How to Get New Dental Patients with the Power of the Web

INCLUDING THE EXACT MARKETING SECRETS ONE PRACTICE USED TO REACH $5,000,000 IN ITS FIRST YEAR

The Ultimate Guide to Internet Marketing for Your Dental Practice

By: Adam Zilko & Jacob Puhl

Disclaimer

The information contained in this book is based on real-life application and factual events, though some names have been changed for confidentiality reasons. We have put forth every effort to ensure that the information is accurate and complete. The information we have presented to you is designed to bring your dental practice all the success it can muster. However, due to variables beyond our control, namely your location and the state of current market conditions, we cannot be held responsible for any loss to your practice after this advice has been put into action. We sincerely hope that this advice works for you and will do whatever we can to help.

If you have any questions, concerns or comments regarding the information contained herein, contact us at your earliest convenience at Admin@Firegang.com.

HOW TO GET NEW DENTAL PATIENTS WITH THE POWER OF THE WEB - INCLUDING THE EXACT MARKETING SECRETS ONE PRACTICE USED TO REACH $5,000,000 IN ITS FIRST YEAR – THE ULTIMATE GUIDE TO INTERNET MARKETING FOR YOUR DENTAL PRACTICE

Published by Firegang Digital Marketing
Copyright © 2014 by Adam Zilko and Jacob Puhl
ISBN-13: 978-1497462700

First Printing: April, 2014
Printed in the United States of America

First Edition: April, 2014

Table of Contents

Part 1:
Dental Internet Marketing – Getting Started

The Story of Mint Dental – How the $5 Million Practice Came to Be

Mint Dental began as many dental practices do. Doctor "J.M." graduated with a Doctorate of Medical Dentistry from Oregon Health Science University in Portland, Oregon and immediately began to fulfill his lifelong dream of opening his very own dental practice. He didn't want to settle in Southern Oregon where he had lived all his life; he had loftier pursuits in mind. So he took his education, training and expertise and opened Mint Dental in the beautiful city of Anchorage, Alaska.

Dr. M. built his practice from the ground up, hired a friendly and professional staff and stocked his office with the latest dentistry tools on the market. To local residents passing by the newly-leased building with the gleaming banner hung over the front door that announced the soon-to-be Mint Dental Grand Opening, here was simply another dentist who seemed to be opening yet another dental practice of which the city already had several to mention. Yet to Dr. M., he was constructing what he hoped would be the biggest and most successful full-service dental practice the city of Anchorage had ever seen.

It didn't take long, however, before the doctor found himself facing a major obstacle.

Inside he had all this passion for providing the local populace with quality dental care using a variety of services from teeth cleaning to IV sedation to dental implants, but, like most dental professionals, he soon realized that he wasn't going to get by on simply being the best dentist in town. Dr. M. also needed to become a business owner; and a darned good one if he wanted to remain a permanent fixture in the local area landscape.

The good doctor of course advertised in the yellow pages, on the radio and did what he could to make sure word-of-mouth always rang positive, but it soon became obvious that all of that wasn't enough.

From day one, Mint Dental found itself in a digital world surrounded by technologies Dr. M. didn't fully understand. Like most in his profession, he was never taught how to properly market his practice in dentistry school. He certainly wasn't taught how to market his practice on the Internet, and with the world going digital, it was soon obvious that Mint Dental was going to be left behind if the doctor didn't act quickly.

Then Dr. M. called us.

What follows are the exact processes we used – with Dr. M.'s help - to take Mint Dental from brand-new office to a practice that earned $5 million in the very first year with Dental Internet Marketing. If you want the same for your practice, dentist, boss or client, turn the page and let's get started.

Chapter 1: Introduction

When we first sat down to write this book, we began by examining all of the current dental Internet marketing books on the market. We wanted to get a sense of what was out there so that we could offer a truly comprehensive book that could be used to maximize any dental practice, but we also wanted to do something no one else had done before.

See, most of the books that we've come across, in book stores, in libraries and on Amazon, were either written by dentists or marketing organizations, but we couldn't find one that represented the idea that we wanted to present to the world.

Our goal from the beginning was to provide a step-by-step resource that any dental office could use to go from modest beginnings to earning $5 million per year, all thanks to the efforts of Internet marketing. The difference between our book and others of its kind is that ours is a result of the collaborative efforts between dental and Internet marketing professionals. Though some names have been changed for confidentiality reasons, the following steps do and have worked for the dental office presented in this book, Mint Dental, and we are confident that they will work for you.

Whether you own a dental practice, work in one or you are a marketer or consultant for a dental professional, this book will help you navigate the ever-increasingly difficult world of Internet marketing.

How to Use This Book

This book is broken up into three parts. You are currently reading the first part, which represents the mental and physical preparation required for getting the most out of this advice.

The second part discusses the most basic of Internet marketing techniques. The steps presented in the second portion are free or low-cost and can be used by anyone to get results – more phone calls, appointments and loyal patients.

The third part represents the more advanced aspects of dental Internet marketing. These are the more in-depth subjects like search engine optimization, local SEO, keyword generation and paid search marketing.

By laying the book out in a step-by-step form from basic advice to the more advanced aspects of the business, we hoped to provide you with a gradual blueprint that you can follow to ultimately reach your practice goals. In this case, we want you to reach the $5 million milestone that Mint Dental recently achieved as a result of this advice.

We advise that you approach this book in one of two ways. The first one is to read through the book from beginning to end, absorbing and learning the steps as you go. Then, when you have finished your first read-through, go back to the beginning and start putting the steps we have laid out for you into action.

The other way we recommend, especially if you are super-ambitious and ready to get started – and more importantly, ready to see real-life results - is to begin putting these steps into action while you are reading, absorbing and learning.

If you do choose to act now, start with the basic section and only then progress to the more advanced techniques once you have gained more experience. Whatever you do, don't give up. Only with constant and consistent effort can you hope to remain competitive in today's ever-changing and evolving marketplace.

A Word on the Technologies and Tools Discussed in this Book

Writing a book like this is tricky because we are describing technologies, tools and processes that are useful today, but that might not be useful five or ten years from now. Actually, let's be realistic. With the way technology is advancing and the Internet constantly evolving, some of these steps may be rendered useless a week or a year from today. The point is, we will do our best to describe every tool and step we provide you with so that you can succeed despite the current state of the digital universe.

Tracking Results and Return-On-Investment (ROI)

By far the largest benefit to Internet marketing, besides the fact that it will lure in patients from far and wide using computers, smartphones and tablets;

is that you can track everything from the amount of visitors who land on your website to the value amount in dollars the average patient represents over a lifetime. You will also be able to determine where your marketing budget is yielding the biggest returns. In other words, where is your money most paying off and how can you maximize those results?

You will find all of that and more in this book. But let's be honest. Information is great, but like Dr. M. when he first ventured into dental Internet marketing, you are yearning for true results. Let's get to those now.

The Results You Can Expect From Using This Book

More Quality Fee-for-Service Patients: Filling your practice with patients is good, but it's not so good if those patients don't desire to maintain a certain level of oral care and they don't have the money to spend on the premium dental services you offer. The advice contained herein will allow you to get much more out of the lifespan of every patient you earn.

Improved Income: This advice helped Mint Dental go from modest beginnings to earning well over $5 million a year in a very short period of time. Follow these steps and you could be on your way to earning much more than you are right now.

Enhanced Marketing Results: As a busy dental professional, staff member, marketer or consultant, you don't have time to toil away at marketing, Internet or otherwise, for little to no return. The steps in this book get results, period.

Increased Case Acceptance: Your premium services keep your practice earning, and we will show you how to sell more implants, root canals and extractions – all of those services that help your practice grow.

***

5 Myths Most Dentists Make When Approaching Internet marketing

For this Internet marketing advice to work, you will need to get rid of all of your preconceived notions about Internet marketing so that you can start with a blank slate, so to speak. Unfortunately, there are quite a few myths surrounding dental Internet marketing. Here are the top five that we encounter most often.

Myth #1: Referrals Alone are the Secret to Growing and Sustaining a Dental Practice.

The Truth: Referrals are great. They can keep your chair filled for days, weeks and even years, but relying solely on referrals is not the way to go. Waiting for referrals to come in is a passive exercise, as you are leaving the power in your patients' hands to spread the good word. Instead of focusing only on referrals to keep butts in your chair, be active and strive to be wherever your patients are so that you can lure them to your practice in droves.

Internet marketing will allow you to keep tabs on your prospective patients and current patients alike. You can show up on their smartphones when they search for a dentist in their area, you can be present on Facebook, which most people manage to visit whether at work or play, and you will be able to take control of your online reputation; which in turn will lead to more quality referrals.

The bottom line is that word-of-mouth referrals can help, but Internet marketing will yield far better results.

Myth #2: New Practice Marketing Can't Compete with Established Practice Marketing.

The Truth: Unlike the past, where it took years for a practice to establish a reputation in the local community, Internet marketing essentially levels the playing field. With the help of ground-breaking online technologies, you can reach out to your patients wherever they happen to be, you can speak to them on their level and you can remain fresh on their minds without being intrusive.

Why don't they teach you this type of stuff in dental school? That's a very good question. Internet marketing is key if you hope to dominate the digital landscape, and we will show you how to do that quickly, with the proper techniques and the right amounts of effort, whether you are new on the scene or not.

Myth #3: Dental Internet Marketing Takes A Long Time to See Results.

The Truth: Some forms of Internet marketing may take time before you begin to see results. It all depends on your approach and the state of current market conditions. On the other hand, you have dentists straight out of school seeing massive results using the latest Internet marketing techniques.

The sooner you act, the sooner you will be able to take control of your online reputation and the sooner you can start making things happen for your practice. Don't get left behind. Take the first step to dominating your local marketplace, which is to continue reading this book.

Myth #4: A Website Alone is More Than Enough for Marketing a Dental Practice Online.

The Truth: You could have the biggest, baddest website in your local area with flashing lights, photos of picture-perfect teeth and all the bells and whistles that are designed to attract quality patients, but if your website isn't converting visitors into actual leads and patients, it might as well not exist.

The ideal way to create an online presence does begin with a website, but it soon develops into a more elaborate net that is designed to lure and, dare we say, trap only the best and most qualified leads. From your website to your blog to your Google pay-per-click ads, you must put focus into all aspects of Internet marketing if you want to attain your true potential.

Myth #5: Most Internet Marketing Techniques Are Free.

The Truth: There is no such thing as a free lunch. In marketing and in dentistry, that phrase couldn't ring truer. Consider your patients that choose to take the free and easy way out. These are the ones who fail to brush regularly and who don't take the time – or spend the money – to visit their dentist on a regular basis.

Just like you advise your patients if they want a happy and healthy mouth, spend the time – and the money – to ensure that your Internet marketing presence is focused and targeted for true results.

As with anything in life and especially with Internet marketing, you truly do get what you pay for. Free techniques can yield results, but the right amounts of capital focused in the right directions can yield eight to ten times the amount of results, or more.

***

6 Internet Marketing Mistakes Most Dental Professionals Commit Without Realizing It

Now that we've cleared up those misconceptions, it's time to get rid of any bad habits you might have – or might inadvertently adopt – once you put these steps into action. The following mistakes are so commonplace that, even if you are not committing them right now, you could find yourself committing them somewhere down the line. By paying attention to these top mistakes now, you will keep your road to success free of any obstacles. In our experience, that is the best way to approach dental Internet marketing when you are first starting out.

Mistake #1: Changing Tactics Too Quickly When Confronted With New Technology.

Imagine if you will, a patient of yours who orders braces, complaining that his teeth are too crooked and that he's just not happy with them. Eager to oblige, you implant the braces and send the patient on his way, but not before scheduling a follow-up appointment in a week or two.

Now what if, at that follow up appointment, that patient comes to you and says, "Doc, I've been reading about clear braces and, well, clear braces are invisible and will straighten my teeth just as good as regular braces, so I want you to rip these braces off and change them to clear braces."

You of course cater to the patient's wishes, implant the clear braces and send him on his way only to have him return for his follow-up to tell you that he's now been reading about dental implants and, well, he figures, "Why am I trying to straighten my teeth gradually over time when I can just have them extracted and have all new fake teeth put in for a movie star makeover?"

How frustrating would that be? Obviously this is an extreme case, but this type of disjointed thinking is exactly what happens to most new dental Internet marketers.

Dental professionals, marketers and consultants alike are all guilty of jumping from one technique to the next in the hopes that one will produce immediate and substantial results. Just as with dentistry, there are no quick fixes and jumping from technique to technique will only force you to go right back to where you started - at the beginning - instead of allowing your gradual results to produce big changes further down the line.

We recommend that you start with one or two techniques, become familiar with those processes and only then move onto newer and more advanced techniques if you want longer lasting results.

Mistake #2: Relying on Little to No Resources to Yield Big-Time Results.

Many of the techniques in this book are absolutely free, and you are encouraged to start with them until you get the hang of things. Yet don't ignore the paid processes and certainly don't discount the prospect of hiring the experts to handle all the Internet marketing heavy-lifting for you. The more resources you allocate to marketing, as long as the proper research has been conducted, the more substantial your yield will be in almost all cases.

Mistake #3: Delaying Your Marketing Decisions Until It's Too Late.

Don't let this book be another that you flip through and promptly set down, never to think of it again. If you do nothing else, at least develop a website or optimize your current website using the steps we have outlined.

The world is constantly changing around you and the longer you hold off marketing your practice online, the harder it will be to dominate when you finally do decide to put your ambitions into action. You hold the secret to dominating the local Internet marketing landscape in your hands. Don't let that opportunity go to waste and take action right now if you have dreams of bettering your current circumstances.

Mistake #4: Failure to Nurture New Leads.

Dental Internet marketing is designed to keep the phone ringing and new patients coming through your practice door, but the rest is up to you. Some prospects that call or visit will only have a slight interest in becoming a new patient. You must keep up with your new leads and use a few best-practices to retain those leads if you hope to convert them into high-quality patients. This book will show you how to do just that.

Mistake #5: Trying to Do Everything By Yourself.

Whether you are a maxillofacial surgeon, a periodontist or a cosmetic dentist, you are likely busy from morning until closing time effectively managing your business. You can't possibly meet and treat all of your daily appointments while answering emails, updating the website, writing blogs and posting on social media all at the same time.

Delegate responsibility when you can and let the talents and skills of those around you work for the betterment of your practice. Social media savvy staff members can handle the social posting, staff members who like to write can handle the blogs and other responsibilities can be divvied up as necessary to keep business and all marketing efforts churning along like clockwork.

This book will show you what tasks to assign for dental Internet marketing dominance.

Mistake #6: Working with Large Agencies and Assuming the Wrong People are Experts.

As your self-managed marketing levels progress and your results begin to become more substantial, you may begin to imagine what a large marketing agency can do for you. After all, you might think, if you can succeed in making the phone ring all on your own, what if the true experts were behind the wheel? We say - buyer beware. Large agencies won't give you the personalized service your practice needs to survive in today's competitive marketplace.

There are also a lot of snake oil salesmen out there who will promise the world in order to get to your money, only to produce zero or lackluster results. Just as a dental patient will research a potential dentist to ensure professionalism, training and experience, you are encouraged to research any potential search engine optimization firms who promise big results in a short amount of time.

Make sure the organization you work with not only has your best interests at heart, but that the people behind the organization are skilled, experienced and able to walk the walk using some or all of the techniques listed in this book.

***

Now that we have helped you achieve the proper mindset, it is time to get started. If you want to dominate your local online marketplace, you first need to develop a solid game plan. That is what we will help you with now.

Chapter 2: How to Create an Internet Marketing Plan

Just as all dental treatments require a plan, so do your Internet marketing efforts. Your Internet marketing plan will allow you to possess a firm understanding of your local market, practice and competition. You will first need to conduct the proper research, which requires three distinct considerations.

Step 1: Who Are You Marketing To? This is where you identify the radius of your target market, as well as create a profile of the ideal patient who you hope will call or visit in the near future. You will be comprising a list of local areas, such as the town, city, county and names of individual suburbs where your patients may reside, as well as analyzing the local demographics and income levels.

Step 2: What Are You Marketing? A proper plan takes into account the practice, staff, staff training and all processes that are currently in place. In the next section, you will learn how to optimize your practice so as to maximize the results of your Internet marketing efforts. The research you conduct will let you know what changes need to be made and where you can improve your practice for even better results.

Step 3: Who Are You Marketing Against? You will soon learn how to identify all of your Internet marketing competitors, as well as pinpoint where those competitors are succeeding and failing in their efforts to secure more local market share. By understanding the opposition, you will be in a far better position to dominate once your campaign is fully-formed and put into action.

***

Here are those considerations explained a little more thoroughly.

Step 1: Who Are You Marketing To? Steps for Identifying Your Target Market

Geographic Location

Start out by making a list of your geographical area and all terms that would be used to describe it. For example, your list might include the state Texas, the city Houston, the county Harris, as well as the area known as Pasadena to help new patients find you. Your list might be long if you live in a densely populated metropolitan area, or it could be short if you live in a rural area.

Here is a tip that we often use to identify a local area for a dental marketing client. We look to see if the local area has a dedicated Facebook page. That page's fans and followers can then be studied to find out who lives in the local community and how best to market to those individuals.

The Ideal Patient

Create a profile of your ideal patient. Include demographics information, such as income level, educational background, employment and other factors that are important to your practice's goals.

While you are encouraged to base this information off of your current patient roster, a much better avenue to pursue is to spy on the local pool of patients using the latest in social networking. This involves using Facebook, Twitter, Google+ and any other social networks to start searching for your ideal patient using the information you have so far gathered.

If you don't have accounts on those networks, not to worry. We will discuss how to set up accounts on the major networks in a coming section. If you do have profiles, use the search functions that those networks provide and expand on your list of consumer research information. Not only are you looking for details on your ideal consumers, but you should also pay attention to the discussions you come across on those networks to determine if you can glean anything from them.

Pay attention to what your prospects and patients are sharing online, how they talk and what they are saying. Your message will resonate with your audience much more effectively if you can emulate the speech patterns and posting styles of those you come across.

***

Step 2: What Are You Marketing? Steps for Analyzing Your Dental Practice

Goals, Strengths and Services

Start by creating a list of your practice goals and strengths. Write down the services that your practice wishes to be known for. List your office hours, pricing and the overall marketing message that your practice hopes to convey.

Marketing Budget

The next step is to establish your Internet marketing budget. Keep in mind that you can effectively market your practice online for a fraction of the cost of traditional advertising. Many of our clients get better results for every dollar they spend online than they do for every $1000 spent on offline advertising. Later we will show you where your money will be best-spent to get the highest return on your marketing investment.

Practice Staff Analysis

Take a good look at your staff and make a list of strengths and weaknesses that can be utilized or improved upon. It would be wise at this stage to identify staff members who have experience with Internet marketing, as well as those who possess social media profiles of any kind. Doing so will provide you with the double benefit of helping you identify areas where staff may need to be trained in the use of Internet marketing and social media to help all future marketing campaigns flourish while the practice remains busy and growing day in and day out.

***

Step 3: Who are You Marketing Against? Studying the Competition

Using the geographical data and services that you established in the preceding steps, search Google for your direct competitors. Pick the top three results for a variety of searches, click on the links and study the sites and platforms that you are presented with.

Make a list of the URL names (website addresses) of those sites, the services listed and anything else you like and absolutely don't like. Pay attention to the office hours, pricing, locations and service areas listed, the extent of your competitors' Internet marketing efforts and anything else that catches your eye.

Finally, call your competitors up and ask them about their Internet marketing campaigns and overall efforts. What platforms do they use, what do they focus on most and what kind of budgets are they working with? This type of recon work can help you develop a marketing plan that is super-competitive for your local market.

Organizing Your Data

Keep these lists handy, as you will be referring to the information over and again as your dental Internet marketing campaigns develop and progress. Handwritten lists are great, but it is a far better idea to create a spreadsheet that you can organize, access, search and filter; allowing for easier recall and improved understanding of the data you have collected.

***

How to Construct Your First Internet Marketing Campaign – Casting Your Net

Once your research has been conducted, you can begin building your first Internet marketing campaign. Your campaign will be constructed using the information you gathered in the previous step. That information can also be used to further target and hone your campaign over time.

Your campaign will be comprised of the following steps, which should be followed in the exact order as they are listed in this book. Each step is briefly explained, but don't worry; all of these processes are fully covered in later sections.

Remember, start off slowly and only move on to more advanced techniques once you gain more experience.

Basic Dental Internet Marketing – Taking the Initial Steps

This is the section where we will teach you the bare-bones approach to dental Internet marketing. You will learn how to put a web presence in place, as well as how to alert your audience that your web presence has gone live.

- **Construct a New Website or Optimize Your Current Website:** Consider this to be your home base of operations, where you will send most of your prospects once your Internet marketing campaign has been put into effect. Your website will prominently feature your phone number, addresses (both physical and electronic) and an online form, allowing for multiple and incredibly easy methods for contacting your practice. This will make it easy for prospects to inquire about your practice or schedule an appointment.

- **Start Blogging:** With the methods you are about to learn, going from website marketing to blogging is as easy as clicking the mouse a few times and writing the words. We will show you how to create an informative, educational and entertaining blog that draws in new, current and previous patients alike.

- **Build and Develop Social Media Accounts:** Social media provides a free and invaluable resource for connecting with prospects anywhere they happen to be. You will soon learn how to create profiles on today's top social media networks, as well as integrate your social profiles with your website and blog.

- **Add Email Marketing to the Mix:** While social media does a fantastic job of keeping your practice on the minds of your prospects and patients, permission-based email marketing represents an even more intimate means of communication. You will soon learn how to build a list of targeted subscribers, as well as write engaging emails and newsletters that always hit their mark.

Advanced Dental Internet Marketing – Going Deeper

In this section, you will learn how the search engines operate and how you can optimize your web presence to show up prominently in search engine results pages. You will also learn how to put a paid marketing campaign into place, as well as how to diagnose problems to keep your campaigns churning along and constantly performing.

- **Pay-Per-Click Search Engine Advertising:** When you are ready to take your results to the next level, we will show you how to put your marketing budget to good use with an ultra-precise PPC marketing campaign using Google Adwords. With your carefully crafted ads in place, patients and prospects will be more likely to see your ads when using the Google search engine. If you thought the phone was ringing off the hook before, with the steps listed in this book you might want to install another line and hire more staff.

- **Tracking, Troubleshooting and Improving Conversions:** Once your net is cast, the last thing you want to do is sit back and hope for results. This book is all about taking action. You will soon learn how to diagnose, test, tweak and further build on your campaign for even more calls, emails and in-office visits.

***

Right now you are probably chomping at the bit, ready to learn these easy-to-implement steps that will help your practice reach its true potential. But before we get started, we urge you, right now, to look around your office. Take a good look at your staff, your equipment and your day-to-day processes and determine if your practice is actually prepared for the Internet marketing success that you hope to achieve. And that is where we will begin this journey on your road to becoming a $5 million practice. So come with us as we first optimize your practice for dental Internet marketing success.

Chapter 3: How to Optimize Your Practice for Success

When Mint Dental first came to us for help with its Internet marketing campaign, we prepared Dr. M. by first telling him exactly what to say to his staff in order to prepare them for the coming influx of new prospects and patients. We told the doctor to expect more phone calls, referrals and office visits. But we also warned him that, if he failed to train his staff properly and if those individuals failed to take the proper steps, all the leads in the world wouldn't mean a thing if those leads weren't retained.

These steps will help to give your practice the boost and polish it needs to retain clients, maintain appointments and create loyal patients for life.

Many individuals contacting you after your Internet marketing campaign goes live will be calling you on the telephone. Start by training your staff to answer the phone properly. For those natural people-person staff members that work among you, let their gift of gab fly and see what works and what doesn't.

For those staff members that aren't so fluent on the phone, here is exactly how to act and what to say to improve the chances of retaining patients each time a new one calls.

Training Your Dental Staff - Turning Phone Calls Into Appointments

It is important for everyone answering the phone to remember that every time the phone rings, there is usually money involved. Not only will new patients bring more money to the practice, but each subsequent ring more than likely originated from some aspect of your overall marketing campaign - and budget. Patient A may call your practice because he found your phone number on your website, and Patient B may have looked up your practice address on her smartphone before she hopped in to check your office out first-hand.

While your practice loses money for every patient that is not retained, your practice gains money for every patient that is. It is the latter that we want to focus on now.

These are the steps we urged Dr. M. to put in place, and they are the steps we urge you to put in place to keep cash flow in the black and the practice constantly growing and improving.

How to Answer the Phone

You can start getting your staff more phone-ready by implementing the following ten steps. You might want to tape reminders to every phone in the office for ease-of-use and to keep anxiety to a minimum. For even better results, make it a contest to determine which staff members can retain the most patients using their new and improved communication skills.

Answer Within Two Rings

You know those patients who call and secretly hope that you don't answer so that they can delay their appointment just a little longer? It is best not to give those people the chance to cancel in the first place. Pick up the phone as soon as the phone rings and never let it go past three rings for best results, even if it happens to be after hours or during lunch.

Give the Caller Your Full Attention

There are two exceptions to the two-ring rule and this is the first one. If you are not prepared to give the caller your full and undivided attention, let the call go to a carefully prepared voicemail message. Then make sure that you call the prospect or patient back as soon as possible.

Don't Put Callers on an Extended Hold

This is the second exception to the two-ring rule. It will only anger your callers if you answer before the second ring only to put them on hold for longer than thirty seconds. If you must put callers on hold, do it for only a moment or offer to call them back as soon as possible.

Important Practice Information

Staff should be adequately trained to give directions, describe service specials, explain insurance details and provide satisfying answers to the practice's most frequently asked questions; all the various subjects that new and current patients might call about. The fewer times you put patients on hold or transfer them to find the answers to the questions they ask, the better.

Use the Same Greeting

Come up with a practice greeting that all staff members must memorize, such as, "Thank you for calling GenericDental, this is Angela speaking, how may I help you?" Say it with warmth and preferably with enthusiasm in your voice, and make full use of your personality to make the call memorable. This makes callers feel special and truly welcome.

Look Forward to Questions

When patients ask questions about services, insurance or billing, let them know that you are glad they asked that question and that you will be more than happy to provide them with an answer. This simple technique can go a long way, especially if the dental staff member answering the phone has genuine warmth in his/her voice.

Don't Forget to Smile

People on the phone can tell when you have a smile on your face. Something about it translates warmth and friendliness in your voice. Train your staff to smile throughout their phone calls in order to bond with every person who calls.

Have Confidence and Be Assertive

Prospects and patients need to be guided into setting an appointment. If Julie who works at the front desk is not confident and doesn't put a little assertiveness in her voice, the prospect she is speaking to on the phone or in person will walk all over her. On the other hand, if Julie can learn to be nice and professional - but also assertive - and she manages to actually tell the prospect to set an appointment, and even goes so far as to mention a date, the prospect in question will be more likely to schedule the appointment she offers.

Always be Nice

You can be confident and assertive while also being as nice as possible. Keep in mind that most people calling your office want you to be the right fit for their needs. They hope the experience works out. Use this to your advantage by being a caring friend to the person you are speaking to.

Avoid Negative Connotations & Language

This will usually require a lot of practice, as most of us are used to telling patients that they 'need to' do this or they 'have to' do that. For instance, your natural inclination might be to tell your patient, "You need to come in every three months or else your gums will recede and your teeth may fall out." While that may be the case, it is the wrong way to approach a patient that you wish to remain loyal to your practice for years to come.

A much better way to approach clients is to use positive language to get your point across. For instance, instead of telling a patient that she 'needs to' come in, you might say, "Our goal is to provide you with a beautiful smile and healthy gums and it would be beneficial to you to come in every three months so that we can keep your oral health at its very best. We can keep your gums from receding and prevent any tooth loss that can result from it."

Language like this doesn't put patients on the defensive and, as they say, you will catch way more flies with honey. Another thing to keep in mind is to leave out the word 'but' from any conversations. For example, instead of saying, "I would love to provide you with an accurate quote, Mr. Smith, but you will need to receive a full oral health exam before we can provide you with an accurate quote." Instead of saying that, it is better to say, "I would love to provide you with an accurate quote, Mr. Smith. Doctor Guzman can provide you with a full oral health examination first, so that we can adequately diagnose any treatment options that may be available to you." Leaving out the word 'but' and keeping language to 'we can' instead of 'you need to' can go a long way towards improving one's professional communication skills.

Quoting Fees Over the Phone

You never know when you will receive a call from a patient who wants to know the exact price of one of your services. This is a critical time, as the person is likely bargain shopping and you may or may not be the first dental professional on the list. And telling people, "We don't give quotes over the phone," is the wrong answer.

When patients ask for service quotes, the correct answer is to tell them that every fee is different and that a full evaluation and diagnosis will be required first before an accurate 'fee' can be quoted. (You are not quoting prices, you are quoting fees). If the caller persists, say that your goal is to provide the prospect with the best and most personalized care possible, and that you won't want to mislead the person by providing a concrete answer over the phone. Let the prospect know that, since he is unique, the diagnosis he receives and the services he requires will be perfectly tailored for him, thus the fees he pays will be completely one-of-a-kind. Then tell the caller that you would be happy to set up an appointment. Then mention a date.

So, a caller asking for a quote on dentures might go something like this.

Mrs. Turner: "Hello, my name is Belinda Turner and I'm wondering about dentures. How much are they?"

Front Desk Julie: "That's an excellent question, Mrs. Turner, and I would love to provide you with an answer. We can schedule you for a full evaluation to see if dentures are right for you, or if another service might be better. Only then can we provide you with an accurate quote. I would be happy to schedule an appointment. Is Monday April 15th good for you?"

Mrs. Turner: "I'm not interested in any other services and I just want to know how much dentures are, please."

Front Desk Julie: "I understand your concern, Mrs. Turner. I assure you that you will be very satisfied with Dr. Smith's evaluation and the fee he quotes you. Since your fee might be different than someone else's, depending on the size and type of dentures you need, for example, it would really be better if you came in to see Dr. Smith personally. We would love to meet you in person. Can I put you down for the 15th?"

Notice how Julie pushed the evaluation and appointment with a specific date each time. That's called closing the deal and every person who answers the phone must be a (firm but nice) closer if you want to enhance your conversions, no matter what callers may be inquiring about.

3 Phone Scripts for More Patient Conversions

The above is a hypothetical conversation that may occur, but the following instances will definitely occur. These are the phone scripts your staff members are encouraged to use to handle the conversations that most commonly take place at dental offices of every type all over the country. These include the new patient phone call, the past-due recall patient conversation and exactly what to say when patients want to cancel their appointments. The goal is to convert these prospects and former patients into actual appointments. Tape these scripts to the phones or keep them in a binder next to each phone and train office staff to use them in order to maximize conversions and minimize cancelations throughout the day.

Remember, these scripts are just a guideline to be used by doctors and their staff, marketers and consultants. After you have gone over them, alter them to fit your own practice needs and then engage in role-playing with your staff members to help their improved phone skills become second nature.

***

The Script to Use When New Prospects Call

This prospect found your phone number online and decided to give your practice a call. Your practice is either completely foreign to him or he may have heard about your practice from someone he knows. In any case, this person is a new prospect and will need to be educated, informed and converted. Here is how it is done.

Staff Member: Thank you for calling **[Office Name]**, this is **[Staff Member Name]** speaking, how can I help you?

Caller: Hello, my name is **[New Patient Name]** and I'm interested in scheduling a teeth cleaning. Do you have any openings?

Staff Member: I'm so glad you called us, **[New Patient Name]**, a teeth cleaning is very important. I would be happy to schedule an appointment for you. How did you find out about our practice?

Caller: I found the website through Google.

Staff Member: That's great news. We sure have put a lot of work into our website. I'm so glad you found us and called. I have an appointment for a teeth cleaning at **[Day and Date]** or **[Day and Date]**. Which one works best for you?

Caller: How much will that cost?

Staff Member: I know that cost is important to you **[New Prospect Name]**, and I would love to provide you with an accurate quote. Before I can do that, **[Doctor Name]** can provide you with a full oral examination to diagnose any health issues before we proceed. Will **[Day and Date]** work best for you?

Tips to Remember When New Prospects Call

1. Call the prospect by name and use language that makes him/her feel special.
2. Keep data mining, but keep it sounding natural by seamlessly inserting data mining questions into normal conversation. Find out how they heard about the practice, what insurance they carry, what oral health problems they face, and so on.
3. Push the appointment and give a choice of acceptable dates to increase the chances of the new patient choosing one or the other instead of denying the new appointment outright.

***

Past-Due Recall Appointments Script

This is often the most feared and stressful phone call that a staff member is required to make in order to keep the practice schedule full. This is the patient who fell off the map. The person may have missed an appointment and has never been seen or heard from again. Getting these types of patients to return takes finesse; and using the tips mentioned above can help immensely. To make the process simpler and to keep staff callers less anxiety-ridden, arm them with all the data they need to make a successful call.

The information they are provided with should include the patient name, the parents' names if the patient is a minor, the patient's date of birth, all contact phone numbers, the best times to call, related insurance information, the frequency of appointments, the hygienist or doctor the patient prefers (if applicable), as well as each date the patient has been seen. Staff should also be provided with the date of the appointment the patient in question happened to miss.

Armed with this information, staff callers need only follow the script, which can go as follows.

Staff Member: Hello, Mrs. Turner, I'm so glad I was able to reach you today. This is **[Staff Member Name]** with **[Office Name]** and our records show that your last professional teeth cleaning and oral health exam was back in March. We want to make sure that you are getting the follow up care that you need. I have two available appointments, one on Monday November 3rd and one on Tuesday November 18th. Which one would work best for you?

Mrs. Turner: Oh, yes, I completely forgot. I've just been busy.

Staff Member: I completely understand, Mrs. Turner, by the way how did your vacation to the Bahamas go? I remember that you said you were going on a cruise.

Mrs. Turner: Why, yes, I did go on a cruise. I'm impressed that you remember that. Put me down for November 3rd. I'll see you then.

Tips to Remember When Calling Past-Due Patients

1. Smile and let the patient know that you care about their oral health.
2. Mark personal details in every file so that they can be recalled when necessary to make patients feel special and remembered, such as asking how someone's previously-mentioned vacation went.
3. If patients want to be called back, ask what time is ideal for them and mark it on the schedule to call back precisely at that time.

***

Script for Patients Who Want to Cancel

When a patient calls to cancel, it is a natural reaction to want to shame the person into recanting their request. We might say something like, "I can cancel your appointment, Mrs. Turner, but you know Dr. Gonzales told you that you need to keep up with your root scaling or else your gums could suffer more damage. You wouldn't want all your teeth to fall out, would you?"

Don't do that unless you want to get hung up on or lose a patient for good. Instead, when receiving a call from a patient who wants to cancel, do your best to help the patient keep the appointment.

If all else fails, reschedule the patient at least six weeks out. This forces patients to act now so that they don't have to wait another six weeks to receive the oral health care they need.

For better results, let the patient know that you don't have any openings at this time, but that you will call back if any schedule changes occur. Then call back in a day or two to offer an appointment six weeks out. Never let patients know that your schedule is wide open, even if it is.

A typical cancellation call might go like this.

Caller: Yes, hello, my name is **[Current Patient Name]** and I'm not able to make my appointment today.

Staff Member: I'm sorry to hear that, **[Current Patient Name]**. **[Doctor Name]** was so looking forward to seeing you today. Is there anything I can do to help you keep your appointment?

Caller: No, I had an emergency come up and I'm just not able to. Can I reschedule for tomorrow?

Staff Member: I would love to schedule you for tomorrow. Our schedule is completely booked up. I can call you back if something opens up.

[At this point, the staff member should call the patient back in a couple of days to let them know of an opening that just occurred six weeks from now.]

OR

Staff Member: I would love to schedule you for tomorrow, let me look. **[Current Patient Name]**, it appears that all of our appointments are booked and confirmed for tomorrow. Our next opening isn't for another four months from now. That's a long time to wait. Are you sure there isn't something I can do to help you keep your appointment with **[Doctor Name]** today?

Tips to Remember when Receiving Cancellation Calls

1. There are no 'cancellations' in the office, only changes and opportunities.
2. Let the patient know that the next opening on the list won't be anytime soon.
3. Try your best to help the patient keep their original appointment.

***

Collection Script

You will grow your practice significantly faster if you can manage to collect all outstanding balances. These are the amounts that may be holding you back from achieving your financial goals so they should not be ignored. The following collection script will help you recoup those balances. The script should be read with a firm yet gentle voice. Keep in mind that you are not calling to collect a payment; you are calling to remind the patient about a charge on their account. As far as you are concerned, the outstanding balance is nothing more than a misunderstanding. Treating the situation this way will minimalize any tense standoffs that can usually occur with calls of this nature.

Staff Member: Hello, may I speak with Mrs. Turner, please?

Mrs. Turner: This is she.

Staff Member: Good morning, Mrs. Turner, this is **[Staff Member Name]** with **[Office Name]**. I'm sure it was just an oversight on your part and I wanted to notify you so that you were aware of it. Our records show that you have a balance of $297 on your account. I would love to bring this current for you. As a convenience, we can put it on a Visa or MasterCard. Which one would you like to use to settle that amount today?"

[At this point, the staff member should remain silent. Silence is a very powerful tool that forces the customer to react.]

Mrs. Turner: I wasn't aware that I had a balance.

Staff Member: Oh, don't worry about it. I'm sure it's just a mistake. It happens all the time. The payment is for the **[Name of Service]** that you received on **[Day and Date]**. We can bring it current right now. Which card would you like to use?"

Mrs. Turner: Yeah, I just forgot. I'll send a check.

Staff Member: Thank you, Mrs. Turner! That sounds perfect. I will put you down for a check to be received in our office by this Friday. Thank you for taking such quick action and we look forward to receiving the payment. I also see that we have you down for March 3rd. I look forward to seeing you. Have a great day!

Tips to Remember when Making Collection Calls

1. Be firm but nice and smile to keep the patient at ease.
2. Let the patient know that it was all a mistake and that it happens all the time.
3. Let the patient know that any future arrangements will be marked down in their file or in the computer, and thank the patient for taking such quick action.
4. Always end phone calls by reminding the patient of their upcoming appointment.

***

How to Respond to Emails and Online Form Queries

Assign staff members to respond to all practice emails in a timely manner. Your website should also include a form that allows prospects and patients to schedule an appointment or contact the practice for additional information. We will show you how to do just that in a later section. For now, prepare your staff for those emails to arrive.

When responding to email, it is important for staff to get the prospect's name, phone number and any other important details they can glean so that a follow-up phone call can be initiated. Email is somewhat intimate as a communication medium, but it doesn't hold a candle to the phone call or in-person meeting. The ideal situation is to get prospects on the phone or in person as soon as possible so that you can connect with them using the human element. It is that very element that will convert prospects into paying and loyal patients.

***

In-Office Visits – How to Meet and Greet New and Current Patients

Your staff should greet every person who walks through the door with an enthusiastic smile. Use the person's name if it is known. If all representatives are currently assisting someone and another prospect or patient walks through the door, staff should acknowledge the person with a friendly nod and let the person know that they will be helped in a moment.

For better results, offer the person coffee and ask them to please make themselves comfortable in the waiting room. Just don't make them wait too long.

When new prospects are finally helped, it is important to greet the person in a friendly manner and to use their name when addressing them. Ask how they heard about the establishment, allowing you to track where the person came from. If the person was a referral from a current patient, make a note to thank and reward that patient somehow.

The overall goal is to make the new patient feel special and to positively reinforce their decision to walk through the door. Make them feel as though they have come to the right place, that their search for a quality dentist is now over and that they are a special and welcome new edition to your dental office. If you can manage to convey those sentiments to every new patient who walks through the door, those individuals will be more likely to tell others of their positive experience.

A typical in-office visit may go something like this.

New Prospect: Hi, I've never been to your office before and I wanted to make an appointment.

Staff Member: That's terrific, I'm so glad you chose **[Office Name]**. What's your name?

New Prospect: My name is **[New Prospect Name]**.

Staff Member: It's great to meet you, **[New Prospect Name]**! My name is **[Staff Member Name]** and the doctor's name is **[Doctor Name]**. How did you hear about us today?

New Prospect: My friend **[Referral Name]** told me.

Staff Member: Well, we are glad to hear that. We really love **[Referral Name]** and I'm going to make a note right now to thank her for bringing you in. I take it you want to schedule an appointment for a full oral exam and teeth cleaning. Why don't we begin by having you fill out a new patient information form? You can sit right over there and enjoy a hot cup of coffee while you fill it out. Here is the form. Please take your time and let me know if you have any questions.

An in-office visit may also go like this.

New Prospect: I'm looking for a new dentist and I've heard about this place. What do you charge for teeth cleaning?

Staff Member: Well hello! I am so glad you chose **[Office Name]**. What's your name?

New Prospect: My name is **[New Prospect Name]**.

Staff Member: It's great to meet you, **[New Prospect Name]**! My name is **[Staff Member Name]** and the doctor's name is **[Doctor Name]**. You said that you heard about us. How did you hear about us specifically?

New Prospect: I looked it up on Google, I think.

Staff Member: Well, we are very glad you did. We have put a lot of effort into our Internet marketing presence to make sure that everyone sees how committed we are to professionalism, and treating our patients with the very best in oral health care.

Now to your question. I'm glad you asked and I will do my best to answer that. The best situation is to have you meet **[Doctor Name]** so that he may provide you with a full oral health exam. Since your smile is unique, your teeth cleaning fee may be different to another patient's. What dental insurance do you have?

New Prospect: I don't have insurance.

Staff Member: Great, less paperwork to fill out. Let's have you meet with **[Doctor Name]** as soon as possible. Why don't we begin by having you fill out this new patient information form? You can sit right over there and enjoy a hot cup of coffee while you fill it out. Here is the form. Please take your time and let me know if you have any questions.

Tips to Remember When Greeting New In-Office Visits

1. Always greet the person by name and acknowledge their presence, even if you are currently helping someone else.
2. Ask how the prospect heard about the practice in order to track marketing results.
3. Get the person to fill out a new patient information form.
4. Remember to ask about insurance and to ask the person to bring proof of insurance to their very first appointment.
5. Schedule the appointment immediately. Everyone who comes into the office – prospect or patient – should have an appointment set sometime in the future.

***

How to Nurture New Leads

Prospects who call, email or step foot into your office are interested in your practice, that much is true; but not every prospect who shows interest is ready to commit. This is where lead nurturing comes into play.

The trick to nurturing your leads is to contact them the moment they show interest and then to stay on top of them until they commit. We are a fan of ranking practice leads according to their levels of interest.

For example, a prospect with a ranking of 1 is not interested at this time, a ranking of 2 indicates that the person is somewhat interested, a 3 is very interested and so on. During your regularly scheduled meetings with your staff, go over your leads, discuss any new prospect details and alter their rankings accordingly. Then schedule your leads to be called so that every morning a certain number of individuals must be contacted and closed.

The following script assumes that the prospect left a voice mail message and expressed great interest in the practice, explaining that he is looking for dental services for him, his wife and his three daughters.

Staff Member: Hello, may I speak to John Strauss, please?

John Strauss: This is John.

Staff Member: Hello, John! My name is **[Staff Member Name]** with **[Office Name]**. I wanted to thank you for leaving a message with our office. I understand that you are looking for dental services for your family. We are so glad you called. How did you hear about us?

John Strauss: I saw the video you posted on Facebook.

Staff Member: Oh yes, our Facebook video. We had a lot of fun filming that video. I'm glad you saw it. And it just so happens that I have the perfect appointment for you. Actually, I have two. You can bring your family to meet **[Doctor Name]** on Monday, December 8th or Monday December 15th. Which one works for you?

Phone Conversions

Have your staff keep track of the number of phone calls that come in and the number of prospects that are closed. Then divide the number closed by the total number called to get your phone conversion rate.

For example, if your staff called 100 people in the span of three months and only closed 29 of those, your phone conversion rate would be $29/100 = 29\%$.

You will be hearing a lot about conversion rates as these lessons progress. Record these conversions and check them regularly to ensure that your Internet marketing and lead nurturing efforts are paying off.

Tips for Nurturing Leads

1. Call leads as soon as possible. Shoot for 24 hours or sooner for best results.

2. Rank your leads according to interest level and keep on top of leads that seem the most ready to commit.
3. Train staff to set aside time to nurture leads every morning.

***

Offline Reputation Management – Word of Mouth & Testimonials

The above steps that outline how to answer the phone, greet customers, retain no-shows and collect overdue revenue will all help your practice improve; and when that happens, word will travel.

To encourage even more patients to spread the good news about your practice and to give them plenty of terrific stuff to talk about, here are the steps we advised Mint Dental to follow as we put their Internet marketing campaign into action.

Steps to Improve Word-of-Mouth & Enhance Testimonials

1. **Train Staff to be Friendly and Attentive:** With improved phone and interpersonal skills, prospects and patients will feel invited and welcome.
2. **Put Some Personality Into It:** Let your inner selves shine to make your office experience even more memorable than it already is.
3. **Explain Everything to Patients in Great Detail:** Strive to help patients understand their diagnoses and the treatments that are recommended for them. Billing and insurance should also be explained. The rule is: the patient should never feel as though they have been surprised or tricked when visiting the dentist.
4. **Provide Amenities to Enhance Comfort and Well-Being:** A cozy waiting room with soft seating, magazines to read, TV to watch and tablet computers to use during treatments are all amenities that can help patients feel at home and ready to boast about your practice with anyone who will listen.
5. **Available Treatments and Quality of Services Rendered:** The fewer times patients have to be transferred to specialists and the more satisfied they are with the services they experience, the better. Word-of-mouth will surely travel if patients can feel confident that the state of their oral health is always in good hands.

6. **Patient Fees Match Perceived Value:** Work to ensure that the fees you charge match the value of the treatments that patients are paying for. In other words, patients should never feel as though they've been overcharged or ripped off if you wish for them to remain loyal.

Testimonials for Marketing and Practice Improvement

We are going to show you how to use testimonials all throughout your Internet marketing plan, but first you have to earn them. We suggest that you get into the habit of asking patients for testimonials following every appointment. Don't just hand patients a blank comment card and tell them to leave their thoughts. That is a good way to get a whole lot of one-word and one-sentence reviews that won't necessarily succeed at showing your practice in the very best light.

Instead of blank comment cards, we recommend that you hand them a card with a series of short but very specific questions on it. This will give them good ideas on what to write about and it gives your practice a good opportunity to study and listen to your local market.

When reading the testimonials that come in, keep in mind that while good reviews are always good, don't become offended if you get a few negative reviews. If you want to know precisely where your practice is weak and where you most require improvement, ask your patients what they really think about your practice and you will soon find out. You can then work on repairing any perceived flaws to improve your practice, reputation and the results you receive from all of your marketing efforts, both online and off.

Sample Testimonial Form

Provide this testimonial form to every patient following every treatment. It is recommended that you supply patients with an anonymous drop box, just in case someone doesn't want to tell you what they really think if the staff happens to be watching.

Dear Valued Patient,

Here at GenericDental, we work hard to provide you with the level of service you deserve. From helping you achieve optimal oral health to repairing your health problems to making you feel welcome and comfortable every time you visit our office, we hope we succeed in making you feel like a valued member of our dental family.

To help us continue to constantly improve, we ask that you fill out this short survey to give us your thoughts, suggestions and honest reviews.

1. What originally led you to our dental practice?
2. If it was due to a dental-related problem, how long had you experienced this problem and how have we done to solve your problem?
3. What three things do you like most about our practice, products and services?
4. What would you tell someone else about us if you knew that person was actively looking for a dentist?

Testimonials should be discussed with the staff on a regular basis, preferably during weekly or daily morning meetings. Let staff know where the practice needs to improve and seek to satisfy those patients who don't seem as happy as they should be.

Your best testimonials can then go on your website, which is where we will now begin your first foray into dental Internet marketing.

Part 2-
Basic Dental Internet Marketing
-Taking the Initial Steps

Mint Dental Ventures Online to Find Quality Patients

With the staff fully-trained and optimized, and with the proper market research conducted, Mint Dental's website went live not long after the practice first opened its doors to the public. The office name, phone number and address were distributed across dozens of online directories, social media profiles went active on a number of popular platforms and a regular newsletter was established. With his Internet marketing net cast, Dr. M. was instructed to go about his business as usual and to prepare for the phone to start ringing.

A few hours after the site went live, the phone began to ring; and it didn't stop. Locals to the area were so intrigued by this new doctor and dental practice that they took to the Internet in droves to search for the office phone number; and pick up the phone they did. They also emailed. Some found the email address on the website, some sent messages via an electronic form on the website and some found the email on one of those aforementioned online directories.

What surprised Dr. M. the most, however, was the number of walk-ins the practice experienced. The practice address could be found everywhere online with a computer or mobile device, and that was no accident. The result was a constant influx of traffic that put the staff's improved training to excellent use.

Almost immediately, the practice began to grow at a stellar rate; and with word-of-mouth ringing positive and online reviews constantly flowing in, Dr. M. was pleased to notice that he was well on his way to achieving his professional goals.

Now you are set to be on the same course.

If you want to establish an online presence for your dental practice that causes the phone to ring, your inbox to fill up and more walk-ins to come through the door than you have experienced before, put the following advice to good use. What follows are the exact steps we took to achieve those stellar results for Mint Dental and now they are about to work for you.

Chapter 4: Construct a New Website or Optimize Your Current Website

Your practice's website is designed to showcase your practice and all that it offers. It should be easy to navigate and contain all the information potential, current and former patients might desire, such as your phone number, the aforementioned practice address, your email address, information about the practice, its staff and doctors, as well as all details regarding all of your dental services.

Your website is so important that you should think of it as your home base of operations or the center of your Internet marketing net that you will cast far and wide to bring qualified leads your way. We are going to show you how to construct a website for your practice that actually performs for you. That is, it will cause the phone to ring and your lobby and inbox to fill up with quality prospects and friendly patients.

If you already have a website, we will show you how to transform that website to improve conversions and leads. That brings us to a very important point.

Your Website Must Drive Conversions

Earlier we spoke of conversion rates when we discussed the process of turning phone calls into patients. Once your new website goes live, you will be looking for other types of conversions, namely phone calls, emails and office visits.

We have already prepared your practice for these types of conversions to take place. You just need to set up a website to deliver them. Here are the steps to follow.

How to Construct a Website

Step 1: Select a Domain Name

Every website on the Internet has a specific digital address, also known as a domain name or URL (Universal Resource Locator). For example, www.Google.com is the domain name or URL of the world's largest search engine.

Before you begin to construct your practice's website, we advise you to come up with a unique website address that will act as your home on the web. The domain name you choose should accurately reflect your brand, be easy to remember and be easy to print on any offline marketing materials your practice produces, such as flyers, business cards and in-office banners.

We advise you to select a domain name that includes your brand name and a word or two that describes your geographical location, such as "GenericDentalOregon.com".

Later in this section we will cover Search Engine Optimization or SEO. These are the techniques that you will soon use to gain favor with the search engines and attract more prospects and patients who may be using computers, tablets and smartphones to locate you.

If you want to gain favor with the search engines with your domain name, putting the geographic location that includes your city and state is a great way to go. Whatever prospective patients might put into Google to search for your practice, those are the terms to consider when selecting a viable domain. Some examples are DentistinAnchorageAlaska.com or CosmeticDentistonMainAustinTx.com.

It is recommended that you select a few domains to choose from, just in case your first few choices are taken. Once you have a list of names, visit a domain registrar of your choice. One of the most popular registrars today is GoDaddy.com, so we will use that as our example.

Visit www.GoDaddy.com (or the domain registrar of your choice) and enter one of the domain names that you just came up with into the search box prominently displayed on the home page.

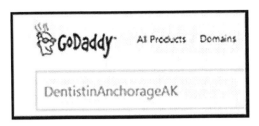

Searching for domain names will let you know which of your choices are taken and which ones are available for purchase. Once you find a name that is available, go through the process of purchasing it.

A domain name can cost as little as $.99 or as much as ten-thousand dollars or more. Play around with various domains until you find a name and price you can be happy with.

When choosing the domain extension (.com, .org, .net, etc.), we recommend selecting .com, as that is the extension that most people know and trust. You can still succeed with a .net or .org, but a .com is far more credible.

You will be asked to select domain protection, which protects your personal information, and a host of associated products, such as email addresses and website builders. For our purposes, you only need a domain for now. Select the options that suit your needs and move on to the next step.

***

Step 2: Open a Web Host Account

In order for your website to be seen, your actual site and all of its documents, images and data files must be hosted on a dedicated server. If you don't have a server of your own, you will have to rent server storage space from a third party. This process is known as opening or purchasing a web hosting account.

You may have noticed that your domain registrar also offers web host accounts. We recommend that you choose a separate host from the domain registrar you have chosen. Some good examples of web host providers include HostGator and BlueHost.

These providers offer excellent customer service and a range of inexpensive product options. Generally speaking, a basic hosting account will run you around $10 per month; or less, depending on the options and time commitment you select. Keep in mind that you will typically have to pay the annual rate up front. Search around for a good deal on basic web hosting service, as web hosts often boast rock-bottom promotion specials.

Choose the host that best suits your needs, along with any upgrades (you won't need any for these purposes), purchase a hosting account and install WordPress.

***

Step 3: Install WordPress – Your Content Management System

WordPress is a universal website-slash-blog creator. It contains all of the capabilities and customization options that webmasters can use to create web presences that range from simple websites with eight-to-ten pages to elaborate sites and blogs with hundreds of pages or more.

There are many benefits to using WordPress to design your site and many companies rely on the system to provide their websites with the functionality they need to impress their website visitors. According to recent reports, the platform is responsible for powering nearly 15% of the top one million websites and nearly half of the top 100 blogs. Though WordPress isn't the only content management system (CMS) available, it is easy to install and implement, so it is the one we are going to teach you how to use right now.

Installing WordPress on Your Hosting Account

We are going to use HostGator as an example of how to install WordPress on the web server space you just rented in the previous step. Once WordPress is in place, you can start creating your website's individual pages and blog posts, as well as manipulate its appearance and functionality.

If you aren't using HostGator as your host provider, refer to your provider's documentation for installing WordPress, or contact a customer service representative to get walked-through the process. Most companies today offer terrific customer support and they will have you set up and ready to develop your site in as little as twenty minutes.

For our purposes, once you have aligned your new HostGator hosting service with your new GoDaddy domain name, visit your HostGator control panel or CPanel.

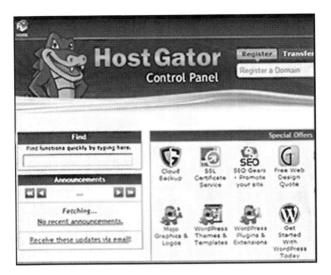

Right in the first section marked Special Offers is a button titled Get Started with WordPress Today. Click that button and you will be whisked away to the WordPress quick install page.

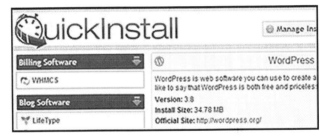

You will be asked to choose the domain name you wish to install WordPress on (you should only have one at this time), as well as a number of other questions. Enter your email address, your website's title, the name of the administrative username you wish to use, as well as your first and last name when prompted.

Click 'Install Now!' and you are finished. You will be provided with your username and login password that will be used to access the dashboard of your site for the very first time.

The WordPress dashboard is where the magic happens. It is your administrator panel, where you will create and edit pages; develop blogs, upload media and all the rest that goes into constructing and maintaining your website. More on that in a moment.

For right now, type your new domain name into the address bar of the web browser of your choice so that you can see how your website looks at this time. Keep in mind that it can take up to an hour or more for your site to appear if you have only recently purchased your domain name. If everything looks good, and you enter your domain name into the address bar of your favorite browser, you should see a Hello World screen, which is WordPress's default design or theme.

To log into your WordPress dashboard so that you can start building your new website, enter your domain followed by /wp-admin/, such as www.GenericDental.com/wp-admin/. You will be taken to the WordPress login screen, where you will be prompted to enter the username and password you were provided with immediately following installation.

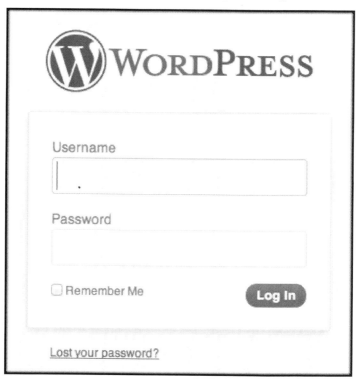

***

Step 4: Customizing WordPress to Suit Your Needs

Once logged in, you will be taken to your WordPress site's dashboard, where the magic happens. For right now, click on the Settings button, which is located in the menu pane on the left hand side of your screen.

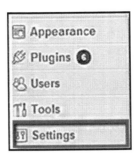

These next few steps will get WordPress customized and ready for you to build your site. First, we need to establish your Home Page.

The Home page is the main page of your site and usually the first page visitors will see when they land on your site for the very first time. Since WordPress was originally designed as a blogging platform, the default Home page is set to show the most recent blog post you have published. Since we want a static or permanent Home page, we need to make a slight adjustment to the WordPress Settings.

Under Settings on the dashboard, find the subheading marked Reading Settings and select A Static Page – Home. This will select your soon-to-be home page as the first page visitors will see when they land on your website.

Next, we want to make your website very friendly to both visitors and search engines by making your website's URL nice, neat and organized. Ideally, you want the website and page name to show up in your visitors' browser address bars when they view particular pages on your website. For example, if they are viewing the Tooth Implants page, they may see a URL that looks like this.

www.GenericDental.com/tooth-implants/

WordPress will allow you to alter the URL of your pages and blog posts whenever you create them, but you can make the process easier by telling WordPress to default to the URL structure that you desire. To do this, select Permalinks under Settings in the left hand pane and then select Post Name under Common Settings.

This will list your domain name followed by the individual page name in your visitors' address bars, just like our example above. This makes your pages easy to bookmark, remember and find. Providing a well-organized site structure also gives the world's major search engines the information they need to rank your pages prominently for all relevant searches.

Step 5: Structuring Your Website

Your website structure refers to the individual pages that comprise it. We advised Mint Dental to structure their website around the practice's services, starting with their site's Home page, which is represented solely by the domain name. There is no extension after the home page, in other words, like so.

www.GenericDental.com

And because of the Settings alteration that you just completed, the rest of your pages will include your domain name followed by the page name, as follows.

www.GenericDental.com/about
www.GenericDental.com/services
www.GenericDental.com/services/dental-implants
www.GenericDental.com/services/tooth-extractions/
www.GenericDental.com/services/endodontics/

In the same spreadsheet that you used to compile your research information, make a new tab and write down the names of every web page that your practice should have; and next to those names write down the coinciding domain names. We will discuss these pages in further detail in a moment.

***

Step 6: Install WordPress Plugins

A plugin is a module that can be installed within WordPress to enhance the platform's functionality. The first plugin that we recommend you install is an SEO plugin.

SEO Plugins

Later in this book there is an entire section dedicated to appeasing the search engines, primarily Google, so that you can put your dental Internet marketing campaign in front of all relevant search users.

Your website will get a head start with the major engines by the settings you have just established and for the inherent fact that your site is built on WordPress. Now you are going to take search engine optimization (SEO) a step further by installing an SEO plugin.

An SEO plugin will give your site and every page you create a boost in the results of relevant searches. The following plugin will help the major engines decide what is relevant and what's not; at least until you learn more about SEO to really ramp-up your results.

How to Install Your First Plugin

We will now teach you how to install the All in One SEO plugin. Keep in mind that we do not endorse this plugin in any way. It comes highly rated and is used by many marketers all over the world, but that could change at any date. We encourage you to use this information to do your own research, read online reviews and find an SEO plugin that is perfect for you. The steps for installing the plugin will be the same, no matter which plugin you settle on.

First, find the Plugins button on the menu pane on the left hand side of your WordPress dashboard. This will take you to the Plugins page.

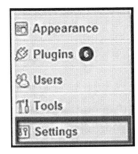

Then click on Add New near the top of the page.

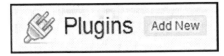

Here you will be presented with a search box. Enter into that box the name All in One SEO Pack.

Notice how there are many listings for SEO plugins. If All in One isn't listed, choose one that you feel will give you the functionality that you need. Otherwise, click on the All in One listing to select it.

Click on Install Now under the All in One listing and, when WordPress reports that the install is successful, click on Activate Plugin. You should now see a button in the left pane of your dashboard that reads All in One SEO.

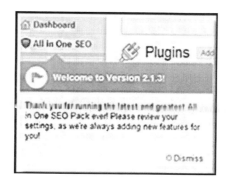

Click on that button and you will see an entire range of options for further optimizing your website for the search engines. You might be happy to know that you don't have to touch a single thing to be optimized for the search engines. Though you can further optimize All in One, the plugin's default settings are more than enough to give you an edge online.

Now that your site's infrastructure is established, it is time to polish up the face of your website, the part that new visitors will see when they land and make their first visit, as well as the functionality that will make your site truly unique.

***

Step 7: Installing Your First Theme – Web Design 101

As we mentioned earlier, the WordPress theme you select determines your website's look, feel and functionality. Your WordPress website comes with a very basic theme installed by default, which you have already seen if you have viewed the Hello World page that acts as your site's current Home page. To make your site one-of-a-kind, you are encouraged to select a different theme before you begin developing your individual pages.

To select a new theme, select Themes under the Appearance button in the left hand pane of your WordPress dashboard.

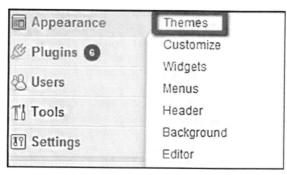

Here you can customize your current theme or select a new one. For our purposes, click the tab near the top of the page that reads Install Themes.

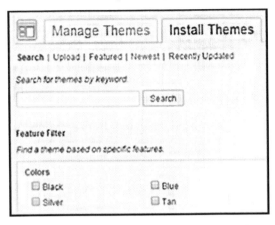

Here you can search for specific keywords or you can view featured themes, newest additions and the themes that have recently been updated. You can also upload themes that you create or find elsewhere.

Free Themes

All of the themes found within WordPress will be free to use as you see fit, but you can also find free themes at sites like WooThemes. If you do a Google search for Free WordPress Themes, you will receive millions of hits, but beware as many of these free offerings are infected with malware, viruses, trackers and other nasties; which makes WordPress themes yet another instance of that old saying 'you get what you pay for'.

Premium Themes

If you want an improved website appearance and extra functionality, you can always find premium themes at sites like Studio Press and Theme Forest. These themes are usually polished and come with fancy bells and whistles like newsletter opt-in forms, message forms, chat and IM boxes; and all sorts of other cool stuff.

Search for a theme that you feel accurately represents your practice and install it using the steps you are about to learn. Once installed, your new theme will instantly go live.

How to Install a Free or Premium WordPress Theme

If you find a theme that you want to use outside of WordPress, under the primary tab Install Themes, select Upload.

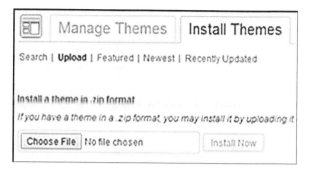

The theme will be in a .zip format. Simply select the file from the appropriate drive when prompted, click the install button and you will be good to go.

All themes can be customized and you are encouraged to customize your themes as much as possible. The ideal situation is to use a WordPress theme that is designed specifically for your practice. You can find professional freelancers for this sort of design work at sites like Elance and Odesk or you can hire local talent by placing an ad in the newspaper or on Craigslist.

The Importance of Web Design

Visitors to your website will begin to judge your website the moment it pops up on their screen. They will decide in that instant if your site looks clean and professional or whether it looks cheap and thrown together. The latter may cause them to click away to choose one of your competitors.

Effective web design unmistakably matches your practice and its overall marketing message. It uses the same colors your practice uses on other marketing materials, the same text font and language; it is easy to become familiar with and remember, and it is considered useful for all who decide to visit.

Your choice of web design is crucial to your overall Internet marketing success. Once you have the right design to match your marketing plan and practice goals, and to make your website truly perform, put these six web design best practices to good use.

1. **Easy to Navigate:** Prospects and patients should have no trouble finding the information they desire. Most WordPress themes are designed to allow visitors to jump from Home to any page on your site in a matter of clicks. To enhance navigation, provide visitors with a menu bar that includes the most important pages with

standard names for pages and a search function. By standard names, we mean not naming your About page Bio, for example.

2. **Simple is Better:** Gaudy websites and sites with too much information jumbled together are typically passed over for simpler sites that don't cause as many headaches when reading. Look at Facebook's design – white background with blue and clearly laid out sections for ease-of-navigation and use. Learn from the pros and keep your web design minimal at best.

3. **Easy to Read:** Choose fonts that are easy to decipher and that look clear on any screen, large or small. Text should be black on a white or light background and should be written in a standard fashion. In other words, write professionally and avoid using tricks to stand out, such as typing in all caps to get your most important points across. Paragraphs should be short and concise with at least a single space between them. Use bullets and bolded subheaders to further break up content and to make the ideas on your webpages easy to digest.

4. **Quality Content:** From the advice you give to the images you use to the videos you film and display, every content element should be considered the best-of-the-best. This is your online reputation we are talking about. Be very selective about what you show to prospective patients, current patients and former patients alike.

5. **Smiling Staff & Patients:** Use plenty of images and videos of happy staff members hard at work and play. Your patients can also be photographed – with their permission, of course – before and after their appointments. Visitors to your site will come away with a much better perception of your practice and your abilities if they know that everyone you come into contact with is just so darned happy.

6. **Calls-to-Action:** For your website to perform, you need to instruct your prospects what to do. Put your phone number prominently on every page and tell prospects, "Call Us Today!" Without strong calls-to-action or CTAs, you leave your website visitors' actions completely up to chance. And we are all about taking action because action breeds results.

***

Step 8: Establish a Prominent Z-Pattern

To develop a well-performing website, you should put your most valuable information 'above the fold', which is the area of your website that visitors see first without having to scroll down the page. Recent studies show that the typical website visitor looks for page information in a Z-pattern. They will first look to the top left of the page, then their eyes will travel to the top right of the page, whereby they will promptly divert their eyes to the bottom left before they shoot directly over to the bottom right. This is all above the fold, mind you.

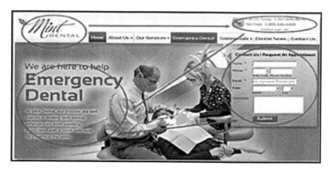

This Z-pattern is where you should list the most important bits of information about your practice so that visitors will see them with a single Zorro-sweep of their eyes. This includes your contact information, special offers, sales pitch, welcome video, contact form and a list of all of the services you want your practice to be known for.

The idea is to give all of your visitors everything they are looking for in a single glance. The less visitors have to work for the information they desire, the more likely they are to choose your practice for their dental needs.

***

Step 9: Reaching Out to Mobile Device Users – WordPress Responsive Themes

Before we get to the individual website pages and what they should contain to enhance conversions, a word should be said about your mobile device-using audience. Back when mobile technology was just beginning to proliferate, it was common for webmasters to keep two sites – a regular one for desktop computers and laptops; and a mobile website for those using much smaller screens.

52

WordPress has found a workaround for this by devising Responsive Themes. We recommend that you use a responsive theme when developing your practice's website. This will automatically tailor your site to conform to any sized screen. Those using desktops and laptops will see your full site, while smartphone, tablet and wearable mobile device users will see an abridged version.

With the help of a responsive theme and the tips found in this book, your Internet marketing message will appeal to visitors, no matter what sized screen they happen to be using.

***

Step 10: Developing Individual Web Pages – Relevant and Useful Content

Visitors arriving on your site are there to find content, which is a broad term that describes the text, images, videos, sound and music files; as well as all the other elements that visitors can see, read, click, hear and watch. For best results, you are advised to populate your website with only the best and most useful information available. Entice new visitors to become leads with engaging content that accurately describes your practice and the services you provide.

You can either write the pages yourself, have someone in your office craft them or you can hire a professional. You can find inexpensive designers, writers, film-makers and other freelance professionals on sites like Fiverr and Tenrr. If you want to get what you pay for, there are always sites like Elance and Odesk.

How to Create Your First Web Page on WordPress

When you are ready to start creating your website's individual pages, go back to your WordPress dashboard and select Add New under the Pages button of your WordPress dashboard.

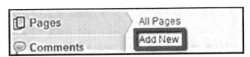

Here you can select your title, write your content, post media and much more. The WordPress page editor is designed to be very user-friendly. If you have ever used a word processor like Microsoft Word, for instance, the WordPress page editor should seem very familiar to you.

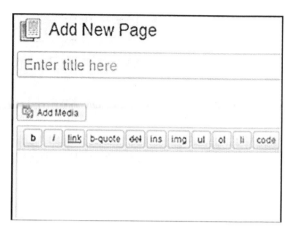

For our purposes, you only need to come up with a title for your page, the content and then click Publish when you are finished.

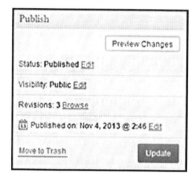

The first page you will create is the first page most visitors will see first; your site's Home page.

The Home Page – A Visitor's First Impression

Your website's homepage is the most important page on your site. As you know by now, it is also the page that most visitors will see first. It must convey professionalism, authority and trustworthiness in a single glance, as well as provide an information-rich Z-pattern above the fold.

Your home page should tell visitors, in mere seconds, who you are, where your practice is located, what they can do on your site and how your office can be contacted. Here are the elements that we suggest if you want your content to truly connect with your soon-to-be-growing online audience.

Contact Information: Most visitors landing on your Home page will be looking for your NAP; your practice Name, Address and Phone number. This information is best served in your website Header and Footer, which are the proper names for the top and bottom sections of your site that remain consistent despite what pages your visitors might be on.

Photos & Images: Photos of your smiling hygienists and clean office – both inside and outside - will help prospects become familiar with your office environment without having to step one foot inside. Use only the highest-quality photos and images to convey the most trust, as well as lend the most credibility to your website.

Contact Forms: To improve website conversions, it is recommended that you give your visitors multiple methods for contacting you. Since your Z-pattern will contain your physical address, email address and phone number, visitors can visit, email or call without needing to scroll or visit any other page. We also recommend installing a contact form on your site, which is a simple questionnaire that captures the visitor's name, telephone number, email address and a short question or comment. Some offices provide an additional line that asks patients to establish a date range for setting up an initial appointment. The fewer questions you ask the better, but contact forms are a must on your Home and all other pages if you want more leads coming in.

To create a contact form on your WordPress site, search for and install the plugin of your choice. Jotform is a good example, but do your own research using the WordPress Plugins search function and choose a contact form plugin that suits your needs.

Most contact form plugins are very easy to customize and they will allow you to create click-ready contact forms in minutes.

Strong Calls-to-Action: Make it easy to contact your practice and tell visitors exactly what to do on every page, such as Call Now, Submit Now, Visit Today, Call to Schedule an Appointment, Fill Out This Form, and so on.

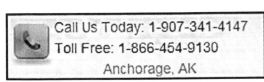

Banners with Sales Messaging: A banner is nothing more than a separate section of your page that showcases your latest treatments and special offers, along with a call-to-action to maximize conversions.

Are you in pain? Broken tooth? Need immediate help?
If you are nervous about   Give us a call today

Dental Treatment   (907) 646 – 8670

We recommend using a banner right on your Home page and above the fold for best results. Some websites have moving banners that alternate between messages the longer someone views the home page. This can be accomplished on your own site by using a Banner Plugin.

Videos: Film under-two-minute videos of your doctors and staff to make patients more comfortable with your practice, and showcase videos of smiling patients to prove to prospects that their oral health is in good hands. Nothing captivates like video. It looks great on your home page and videos can be easily shared on social networks. We recommend you use them whenever possible.

Why Choose Us: We are a big fan of placing a separate section near the bottom of your home page that asks patients Why Choose Us? You can then supply visitors with a short list of bullet points that represent the most advantageous attributes of the service being offered.

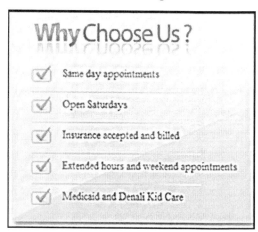

Why Choose Us?

- ☑ Same day appointments
- ☑ Open Saturdays
- ☑ Insurance accepted and billed
- ☑ Extended hours and weekend appointments
- ☑ Medicaid and Denali Kid Care

Testimonials: People like to know that others have enjoyed your dental services before they commit. Make the decision to convert an incredibly easy one for your website visitors by listing your testimonials right on the home page.

Social Media Integration: You will soon learn how to set up Facebook, Twitter and Google+ profiles, as well as a YouTube channel and other social media accounts. Social buttons, which are clickable icons that lead directly to your individual profiles, can then be placed on your home page to show that your practice is active and ready to engage on the world's most popular social networks. You can do this easily by installing the respective Social Media Plugins. Or you may be able to find a comprehensive social media plugin that does the job of several plugins in a single install.

Trust Emblems: This section of your home page is where you will place logos for the Better Business Bureau, American Dental Association and other relevant organizations to lend further credibility to your already professional-looking website.

Search Box: The key to high-optimization is to make your content incredibly easy to search and locate. Putting a search box right on the home page is a great way to ensure visitors can find what they are looking for within a few clicks. This can be accomplished by using a Search Box Plugin.

Photo Gallery: If your theme doesn't come with a photo gallery, you can install a WordPress Plugin that will help you showcase a range of photos in all their glory. Visitors will then be able to scroll through your photos and see them close-up, providing an even more enjoyable user experience.

Footer Elements: The bottom section of your WordPress site, or the footer, represents a valuable area of web real estate that allows you to provide even more important information for your visitors to find. Your footer can contain your practice name, address and phone number (NAP), a sign up box for your newsletter, social media buttons and links to your site's legal and copyright information.

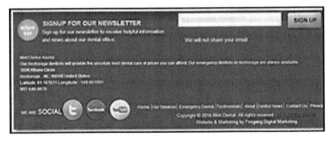

Not all of these elements are necessary, but the more you include – as long as they are organized properly – the more information you will provide and the more conversions should come in. You can make this process simple by installing a Footer Plugin.

***

Step 11: Create the Other Pages that Will Comprise Your Dental Website

About Us – A Chance to Tell Your Story

This is the page prospective patients will visit to learn more about your practice and all the important people behind it. People coming to your About page are expecting to research the dental professionals who run your practice, their levels of education, their experience levels and possibly information about their personal lives.

Visitors landing on your About page may also want to learn about – and view photos and videos of - the dental staff. A good way to present this information is to offer a photo of each staff member along with a short bio, their title or position, their responsibilities and possibly their hobbies, aspirations and dreams.

And don't forget the story of how your practice came to be, why you chose the town you settled in and what the practice's mission statement and goals happen to be.

This is your chance to let your prospective patients know all about your practice and, more importantly, that there are people and personalities behind your quality services; and that all they have to do is email, come in or call to learn more. In other words, don't forget your call-to-action at the end of your About page content.

Services – Your Practice's Money Pages

Your practice doesn't make money off of oral exams and cleanings; it's the big ticket cases that cause the bottom line to jump. Implants, extractions and dentures, oh my. These are the pages that many visitors will be focused on. For this reason, you should strive to answer any potential questions and teach visitors a thing or two while they are browsing.

As we have already mentioned, we recommend that you create a new page for every service that your practice offers, which might cause your URL structure to look something like this.

www.GenericDental.com
www.GenericDental.com/services/
www.GenericDental.com/services/dental-implants
www.GenericDental.com/services/tooth-extractions

Notice how the Services page is a Parent page and the actual services (i.e. Dental Implants and Tooth Extractions) are the Child pages. You can select your Parent pages and their Children in the WordPress Page Edit screen in the same box as the Publish button.

When crafting your services pages, be sure to include before-and-after photos, testimonials and general advice, as well as real-life stories in order to convey your authority and entice more site visitors to convert.

FAQ – Your Practice's Most Frequently Asked Questions

In an earlier section we mentioned taping a list of the practice's most frequently asked questions next to each phone to help staff members become more informative and helpful. Wouldn't it be great if prospects could have all of their questions answered on your website before they call, thus freeing up valuable office resources? This can be easily accomplished by providing a list of questions and answers on a separate dedicated web page titled Frequently Asked Questions or FAQ for short.

Be sure to bold your questions to make them easier to see on the page, and to give your page a nice visitor and search-friendly structure.

Testimonials & Reviews

We spoke of testimonials in the preceding chapter and we mentioned that those word-of-mouth tidbits could be placed on your website. This is your chance to create a page dedicated to the kind words of your valued patients.

In addition to a Testimonials page, we recommend including a Review Us page. In a later chapter, we will discuss review sites like Yelp, Foursquare, Angie's List and others. The Review Us page is a good location to place buttons that lead directly to your profiles on today's most popular review sites. As you will soon learn, people trust review sites online as much as they would a personal recommendation from a friend, relative or co-worker.

Steps to Take When You Already Have a Website

If your current practice's website is not a WordPress site, and you wish to keep the format, apply everything we have just taught you to your old site to the best of your ability.

However, we recommend that you create a new site or at least transfer your old site to WordPress. Simply follow the steps as we have laid them out for you and transfer as much as you can from the old format. Patients who have visited your old site will be sure to take notice and that may be all they need to pick up the phone, email or come in; which is the exact goal of a well-performing website.

***

If you followed the above advice, you now have a fully-functional, well-designed and well-performing website. You have also optimized your site for the search engines, so searchers who are looking for a dental professional in your area should be viewing your site soon.

And now that your website allows for several methods of communication between your practice and all of your prospects and patients, your phone should start ringing, your inbox should start filling up and more prospects should be walking through your office door.

Once you are comfortable with website marketing and only when you think you are ready to move on to the next step should you proceed to the next section of your dental Internet marketing plan: Blogging. And since WordPress was designed to be a blogging platform first and foremost, creating your first blog post is as easy as visiting your WordPress dashboard and clicking Add New under the Posts button in the left hand pane.

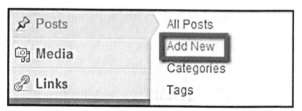

Chapter 5: Start Blogging

If your website's About page was a chance to tell the unique story of your practice, your blog offers the chance to truly embellish. Your blog is also a prime location to discuss the latest changes to your office, the most recent advancements in dentistry and the importance of keeping a clean and healthy mouth.

WordPress allows you to seamlessly merge your blog to your website, which – with enough fresh and useful content – will drive even more traffic to your site and should help to deliver more conversions. Since your WordPress website will provide the infrastructure for your blog, you just have to come up with the useful content.

A blog, short for web log, is typically written in the first person. Its primary design is to allow a person or company to offer their personal viewpoints and to educate others about a particular subject. A dental blog is your chance to put your personality behind your brand. It allows you to establish your authority over your audience and it keeps your prospects and patients informed and educated. And lastly, a blog is a terrific way to keep your website and all of its individual pages and posts in the good graces of the search engines.

Search engines like Google love fresh and valuable content and they will oftentimes rank newly published pieces higher than old and stagnant pages and posts. Keeping your blog constantly updated can improve your search rankings, which can contribute to higher amounts of web traffic and conversions.

Quick Blogging Tips

For a blog that keeps your prospects, patients and the search engines constantly clamoring for more, put these seven blog writing best practices to good use.

1. **Post Often:** For best results, we recommend that you post at least four times per month, or more if you have the time and subject matter to sustain that much content.

2. **Quality Over Quantity:** The exception to the above is that you should only post if you have something valuable to say. It is better to have a few great posts than dozens of mediocre ones.

3. **Proper Word Count:** Studies show that readers and search engines prefer posts that hit the sweet spot between 400 and 700 words. That is plenty of room to tell a story, get an idea across or teach your readers a brand-new lesson.

4. **Check Grammar, Spelling & Accuracy:** Read over your posts once, twice and even three times and give them to colleagues and staff members to read over before they are published online. The fewer errors readers see and notice, the better.

5. **Have a Conversation:** To enhance the bond that you will inevitably develop between you and your growing audience, speak with your readers on their level, and invite them to respond to your thoughts and ideas in the comments section.

6. **Ask for Comments:** One of the hallmarks of a successful blog is a robust comments section. The more comments your posts earn, the more likely new readers are to leave a comment of their own. WordPress makes it easy for readers to comment, but you can get things started by using strong calls-to-action, such as, "Leave a comment and tell me what you think."

7. **Supplement with Eye-Catching Media:** Just like web pages are better served with high-quality images, photos and videos, your blogs will become even more engaging and memorable with the proper and most strategically-placed media.

The Art of Engaging Blog Titles

Starting a blog in WordPress is just like starting a web page. After you click Add New under Posts in your WordPress dashboard, you will be taken to the Post Edit page where, just like in the page edit screen, you will be prompted to insert your new blog post title.

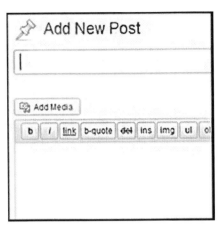

It is recommended that you create several titles for every blog post you plan to write, whereby you will choose only the very best ones from your list to actually publish. The best blog titles are short and concise, edgy, thought provoking and driven by action verbs.

Spend some time studying the top news headlines and the most read and commented-on competitor blog posts and use that information to make your blog titles even more powerful.

Blog Post Ideas to Keep the Fresh Content Coming

We recommend that you create a list of blog subjects that you plan to write about in advance, such as during the time you are developing your dental Internet marketing plan. This will provide you with an end goal to focus on and will leave you less likely to peter out once the initial enthusiasm wears off.

In our experience, many dental Internet marketers – and Internet marketers of every kind – have this burning desire to succeed when they first get into the game. It doesn't take long for that winning attitude to fizzle away, especially when they don't experience drastic and immediate results, and soon Internet marketing begins to feel like work. Without a solid plan, many Internet marketers choose this low point to quit the game entirely.

But you are different. We can feel it. Thanks to our help, you have a marketing plan and your plan should include a long pre-established list of blog subjects and titles. With most of the work done, you just have to fill in the blanks with valuable content and multimedia. No pressure, it only takes focus, a desire to succeed and, you guessed it, a plan of action.

To keep your blog churning along, here are ten subjects to keep your readers on the hook.

1. **Industry/Breaking News:** Show your readers that you are keeping up with the latest goings-on in your industry by acting as a major news source for the dental industry.

2. **Case Studies & Patient Experiences:** New patients will want to know if your services are effective and if they are worth the money they will be paying. Publishing actual case studies and relaying the actual experiences of your patients – possibly even in their own words – will help new patients become more familiar and comfortable with your practice. This is a great way to grease the wheels on the conversion train.

3. **How-To's & Expert Advice:** Show your blog audience how experienced and knowledgeable you are by teaching important lessons, like how to properly care for the teeth, gums and mouth; how best to prepare for appointments and the best ways to recover after major treatments. This establishes you as an authority in your field, thus making you the go-to professional in your local area.

4. **Frequently Asked Questions:** Any new questions that seem to be asked repeatedly should be added to your FAQ web page; but there will inevitably be those questions that you want to provide a more elaborate answer to. A blog post is the perfect medium for just that very thing.

5. **Product/Service Reviews:** Your readers will want to know your practice's opinions on many of the popular dental products and services on the market. They may also want to read honest reviews of your dental services. Don't make your readers wonder what your opinions are. Start blogging and make your opinions known.

6. **Top Lists:** Numbered and bulleted lists are very easy to read and digest; and readers love them. Incidentally, titles with numbers in them tend to perform better than titles without them.

7. **Year in Review & Predictions:** As the year draws to a close, provide readers with a breakdown of what went on within the office and with the practice in general. You can also do your best to predict what will be coming in the next year, discussing such subjects as advancements in the industry or the expansion of your practice.

8. **Debate & Controversial Blogs:** Don't be afraid to go ag public opinion for fear that you will ruffle feathers and lose readers. Blogs that always toe the line are boring to read and they don't get nearly as much traffic as blogs that go against the grain now and again.

9. **Video Blogging:** Instead of writing out every blog, you can film your ideas instead. Most adults these days have smartphones and most of those phones come with top-of-the-line cameras and video cameras built-in. To appease both readers and watchers alike, you may want to supply a written account of the action immediately following every video blog post you publish.

10. **Aggregate Other Blog Posts:** If you are absolutely stuck on what to write about, visit other blogs in your industry and pick the top posts for that week or month. You can then provide links to those blogs along with a note explaining why you chose each post. Google likes it when you link out to relevant content and linking to relevant blog posts is a great way to do it. You will also be showing love to your competitors and you never know when they may return the favor, thus increasing your reader base.

Google Authorship

You have probably noticed that throughout this book we have mentioned several tricks for getting into Google's good graces. Google is the largest search engine in the land so we want to appease that engine first. Once you experience high rankings in Google, the rest of the search engines should rank you prominently by default. Appeasing the search engines is crucial if you want large amounts of visitors to your website and blog.

Yet another trick for gaining favor with Google is to set up Google Authorship within your blog. Google established this markup ability in an effort to determine who was producing the highest-quality content. The markup is connected to your Google+ profile, which is the name of the search giant's social network. This makes it so that anyone who sees your blog posts in the search engine results will also see your Google+ photo and other important information about you, such as a link to more of your valuable content.

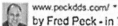

Dr. Fred Peck is a Family and Cosmetic Dentist in Cin...
www.peckdds.com/ ▾
by Fred Peck - in 73 Google+ circles
Dr. Fred Peck, a third generation general dental
professional helping the **Cincinnati,** Montgomery, Mason
along with Blue Ash, Ohio locations is actually

This brings us to the next section of your Internet marketing plan: Establishing a social media presence; where you will be reaching out to your Internet marketing audience in all new ways using today's hottest and most popular social media networks. We will come back to Google Authorship at the appropriate time. Until then, keep publishing high-quality blogs and only move on when you are ready to ramp-up the results your practice should already be experiencing.

Chapter 6: Build and Develop Social Media Accounts

Every bit of advertising and marketing that your practice engages in is about putting your brand as well as all product and service offers in front of viable patients. Social media is one of those rare forms of marketing that enables you to reach out to and connect with your prospects and patients wherever they happen to be.

With smartphones in most pockets, tablet computers in many homes and desktops and laptops in nearly every home and office, more people are connected to the Internet than ever before, and most people today use social networking.

This includes your teenage patients, their parents and even their grandparents. If you were to take a poll of your office staff and every patient on your current roster, you would likely find that 99% of them have at least one social networking account.

To maximize your chances of reaching as many people as possible that live within your local geographical area, we are going to recommend that you start with the three most popular social networks on the scene – Facebook, Twitter and Google+. We are then going to recommend a few smaller social networks to maximize your chances of reaching out to everyone in town.

Step 1: Set Up a Facebook Account

Facebook is considered the best and most popular social network in the world. The platform boasts over a billion users worldwide and it is used by people of all ages from teenagers to the elderly.

Out of all the social networks we will soon mention, it is a good bet that most of your staff and patients have a Facebook page. And according to most studies, both your staff and those patients are visiting Facebook at least once per day, even while they should be working.

To create your Facebook profile, visit www.Facebook.com and select the link near the bottom of the page that reads "Create a Page for a celebrity, band or business". If you already have a personal Facebook account, click on the gear icon in the top right corner and select Create a Page.

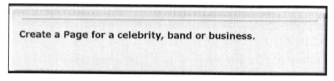

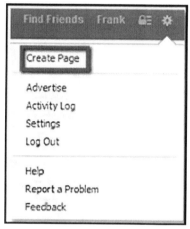

This is known as a fan page. You will next be asked to select the type of fan page you wish to create. To create a dental Facebook fan page, select the option Local Business or Place.

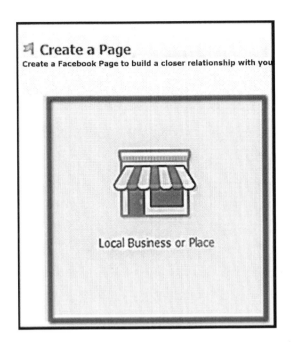

Create a Page

Create a Facebook Page to build a closer relationship with you

Local Business or Place

If you already have a Facebook account and you are not logged in, you will be asked to select your category. We recommend that you select Doctor. Fill out the rest of the information, click on I agree to Facebook Pages Terms (after reading their terms, of course) and click Get Started.

The first step to filling out your Facebook page is to fill out your practice's About information. Select your Categories first. We recommend you insert your profession and the services that you wish to be known for.

For example, you might select Dentist, Root Canals, Teeth Extractions or Full Smile Makeovers. Think of terms that other Facebook users might type into the Facebook search box to find your practice and enter those terms as categories. These terms are known as your keywords, which we will discuss in greater detail in later sections.

Facebook will actually help you select the most popular keywords to use. The moment you begin to type, Facebook will try to predict what you are trying to actually say by offering a list of viable alternatives. For example, if you type 'tee', Facebook will automatically return the result Teeth Whitening. Use these predictions to your advantage by selecting a variety of categories that will expand your reach even further across the Facebook network.

Your description should be a concise summary of your About webpage. Describe your practice, doctors and staff; and use a call-to-action to invite all of your profile visitors to click on the link that you are about to provide.

Enter your website domain or URL into the provided space and select Yes when asked if your practice is a real establishment, business or venue. You will also be asked if you are the authorized representative of that establishment. Select Yes and continue.

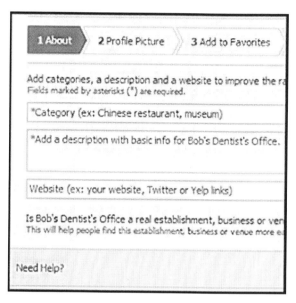

Next you will be asked to upload a photo from your computer or hotlink a photo from a particular website. Choose a photo that accurately represents your practice, such as a group photo of dentists and staff standing in front of the sign out front, or something similar. Make sure it is of the highest quality to put forth the very best first impression.

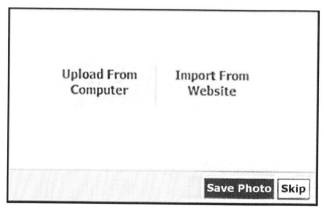

The next two questions are optional. One asks if you wish to have your business page listed as a favorite on your personal account. This is completely up to you, as it is merely a way to make your business page more easily accessible. The next question asks for a payment option for the purposes of engaging in Facebook paid advertising. For right now, you are more interested in free social media marketing and so we urge you to bypass the paid option for now so that you can proceed to the Facebook Admin Panel.

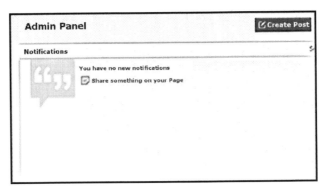

Your Facebook Admin Panel is where the magic happens. Here you can create new posts, upload photos, see who has 'Liked' your page (a Like is a conversion in Facebook) and determine how your page is doing overall.

For right now, just make sure that your photos look good, your information is accurate and that your posts are valuable, consistent and constant.

That's all it takes to get started marketing on Facebook. Here are six steps to keep your Facebook account engaging, up-to-date and converting.

1. **Choose Multiple Administrators:** Facebook allows you to select several individuals who will have administrative privileges over your Facebook account and all of its content. Select several staff members to post on Facebook and instruct them to respond to all questions and messages in a timely manner to keep engagement fresh.

2. **Make Inviting Friends Fun:** Host a contest for staff and patients alike to see who can recommend the most Facebook fans to your page. The winner can receive a gift card and be featured on the website, blog and all other social media accounts for even further reach and engagement.

3. **Remain Interesting:** People check Facebook on their computers and mobile devices when they are bored and they are merely seeking interesting content to keep them entertained. In a perfect world, your Facebook account would constantly post intriguing, thought-provoking, funny, awe-inspiring and tear-inducing content. Be the page everyone has to visit at least once per day and you will have an easier time attracting fans, conversions and leads.

4. **Engage People:** Listen to the conversations your prospects and patients are having and be helpful when you can. Answer questions, instruct and entertain. The beauty of Facebook is that you can get up-close-and-personal with your target audience. Take advantage of that ability by participating in dialogues you otherwise couldn't engage in.

5. **Specials & Promotions:** The next time you offer free teeth whitening, $25.00 oral health exams or a free Invisalign consultation, send a Facebook post to all of your fans. Just a single glance on a screen of any size will implant an idea that could translate into a commitment to call, email or come in at a later date.

6. **Be Visual:** Use your best office photos that successfully promote your dental office and all of your products and services. Studies show that Facebook posts that include photos receive 120 times more engagement than posts with mere text. For best results, post impromptu photos of staff in the office or smiling patients following their treatments.

***

Step 2: Set Up a Twitter Account

Once you have become familiar with Facebook, you are encouraged to move on to Twitter, the world's second largest social network. Whereas a blog is a place to share your extensive thoughts in under 700 words, Twitter only allows you to enter 140 characters at a time. Hence, it is known as a micro-blogging platform.

Many people use Twitter to stay connected and to receive the latest breaking news and information. In fact, many news sources are now citing Tweets (Twitter messages) in their articles, and the Centers for Disease Control (CDC) is even keeping an eye on the platform and its rapid-fire content to help track the spread of major illnesses, like the flu. With the right amount of targeted tweets that are both timely and useful, you can succeed at remaining connected with your prospects and patients anywhere and at any time.

To create your Twitter profile, visit www.Twitter.com and enter your name, email address and an easy-to-remember password when prompted.

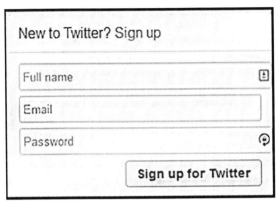

Next you will be asked to select your Username, which should closely match your practice name. Keep in mind that you can always change your username if you happen to think of a better one later.

Select the checkmark Tailor Twitter based on my recent website visits; then click Create my Account.

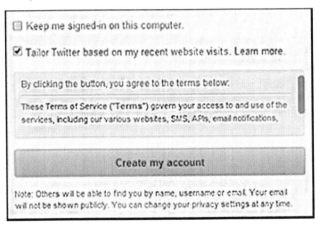

The next few screens will take you through a quick Twitter tutorial. You will learn the true definition and length of a tweet, how to follow other Twitter users – you will be required to follow five or more regular people or organizations and five or more well-known people or organizations to continue – how to add contacts from your various email accounts, how to add a photo and how to enter a bio.

From the colors you choose to decorate your profile with to the photos you upload to the information you provide – it should all be apparent that your Twitter profile is associated with your practice's Facebook page, website and blog.

Once your profile is established, here are five Twitter best practices that will help you get the most out of this growing and incredibly-addictive social network.

1. **The 70-20-10 Rule:** Remember this rule when tweeting: 70% of your tweets should share your webpages, blogs, articles, specials, images and videos. 20% of your tweets should focus on connecting with other twitter users with the hopes of forming relationships. And 10% of your tweets should be about relevant but interesting content – breaking news, actual patient experiences, new treatment offerings, etc. This formula has been shown to attract the most attention on Twitter.

2. **Find Friends & Follow:** Use Twitter's search function to find local prospects, patients and dental professionals alike. Find out who your followers are following and follow those people and organizations for even greater reach. With Twitter, you might be having a conversation with one of your patients or the head of the American Dental Association in the same news feed. Just keep in mind that the ones you follow are the ones whose tweets you will see in your news feed. As you will soon see after getting used to the platform, you will want to be selective of whose tweets you are exposed to.

3. **Tweet Often:** For best results, we recommend that you tweet at least three times per week. You have very few words to convey your thoughts along with any links you wish to provide, and all in 140 characters. Like we recommended with your blog titles, write several tweets and select the best ones to submit. Keep an eye out for your competitors' tweets to get an idea of what your audience best responds to.

4. **Use Your Title-Creation Skills:** Since Twitter only allows a few words to get your point across, you can largely think of it as a title. Use the same advice you used to create your webpage and blog post

titles. Go for concise tweets with lots of action verbs and try to add links to engaging content as much as possible. Remember, your tweets have to drive conversions, which could be a direct message, a click-through to your website or a phone call to your office. Be selective about the things you tweet and always try to help, serve and connect with your audience with every tweet you send.

5. **Ask Questions:** A trick to get more attention to your Twitter profile is to ask a question or stage a poll, such as, "Austin: Do you brush and floss after every meal?" A simple question will force users to want to engage, and you never know what type of conversion that engagement will lead to.

6. **Show the Love with @'s and Retweets:** The 'at' symbol is used on Twitter to reference other Twitter users using their username. One of your tweets might read, "Thank you @AndyParks for referring our new patient @SuzieHanks". And you are encouraged to 'retweet' notable tweets from your followed and followers as they show up in your news feed. There is a retweet button at the bottom of every tweet in your feed to make the process simple.

7. **Use Hashtags (#) When Appropriate:** The pound symbol that we all grew to love has been replaced by the hashtag. The hashtag preceding a term will cause that term to become a separate tweet category in Twitter. Examples include #GenericDentalBDays where you compile all of your patient birthday announcements and #GenericDentalSpecials where you organize your discounts and free offers. All you have to do is tweet a message followed by a hashtag or two like so, "Happy birthday @SuzieHanks from all of us here at GenericDental! #GenericDentalBdays," and Twitter will do the rest. Use hashtags only when appropriate, two only when absolutely necessary and never use more than that.

***

Step 3: Create a Google+ Business Account

If you want Google to favor you in the search results, it only makes sense to create and manage an account on their proprietary social network, Google+. You may already have a Google+ account. If not, we recommend that you create one so that you can obtain a Google email address (Gmail) and password, which we will be using extensively in later sections. For right now, we are going to focus our efforts on the professional platform within the social network, otherwise known as Google+ Business.

Google has changed the name of its local Business network several times in the past few years. First it was Google Places, then it was Google Places for Business and now it's just Google | Business. So you have Google+ for social profiles and Google+ Business for professional enterprises just like yours. We recommend that you create profiles on both networks before you proceed.

While you may not have as many prospects and patients using Google+ as you would using Facebook or Twitter, the network can still expand your marketing reach and you are encouraged to use it. The reasons are a potential boost in the search results and the fact that you can implement Google Authorship, the search engine visibility advantage we discussed briefly in the blog section.

Keep this in mind as you fill out your About information, which Google calls your Story. Then select your profile photo, which can be the same as the profile photos you used on Facebook and Twitter.

The process for setting up and managing a Google+ Business account is very similar to managing your Facebook page, so you should become acclimated quickly.

First visit https://www.google.com/intl/en/+/business/ and click the button marked Get Your Page. Or Log In if you already have a Google+ account.

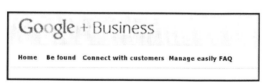

Here you will be asked which type of page you would like to create. Just like you did when you created your Facebook profile, click on Local Business or Place and proceed to the next step.

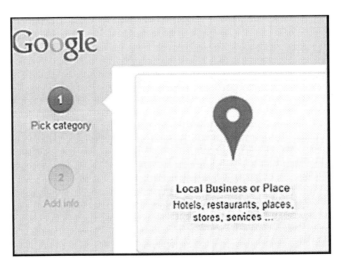

At this point, Google wants to make sure that you are not creating a duplicate page, just in case you already have a Google+ Business page in existence. Google will oftentimes aggregate or pull information that it finds on various sites across the Internet, such as from local yellow page directories. This information will be used to compile a page that you must claim and control.

You can search for a current page by using your practice name and/or address when prompted.

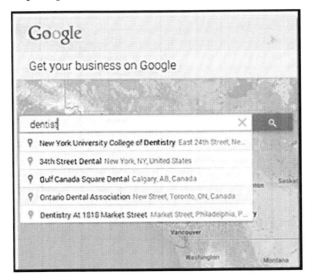

If you don't see your practice name listed, you are encouraged create a new page. Enter your business details when prompted and continue on to the next step.

If your practice does come up when you search, select the listing and claim it. Claiming your page will allow you to control all of the information listed on your Google+ Business page. Furthermore, the act of claiming your page sends Google a message and confirms that the page information is absolutely complete and accurate.

Google allows you to verify your listing by phone or post card. Select the option that is best for you, follow the steps and then proceed to your Google+ Business dashboard.

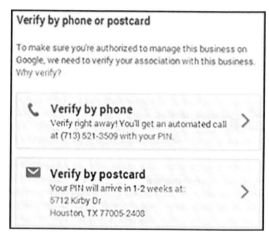

Once you are in your page's dashboard, you will be taken through a virtual tour that will encourage you to fill out your profile, create a new post, set your notification settings and upload a profile photo.

Take this tour and complete your profile using all of the information you used to fill out your Facebook and Twitter profiles. Again, the idea is to get visitors to your profile excited enough about your practice to call, email or come in.

Once your Google+ Business profile is optimized for conversions, you can proceed to your dashboard to post and communicate with your audience.

The Google+ Business dashboard is designed to be very user-friendly. You can send new posts, see how your page is performing or you can implement paid online advertising.

For right now, use these seven Google+ Business best practices to keep new followers and conversions coming in.

1. **Encourage More +1's:** Facebook has the Likes conversion and Google+ has the +1. Ask your staff and patients to visit your page, interact and click the +1 button to experience even more social clout.

2. **Fill Out All Profile & Practice Information:** Don't leave any sections blank. From your story to your practice address to your practice hours of operation, spend the time to ensure the information is thorough and correct.

3. **Build, Organize & Manage Circles:** Google+ makes it easy to segment your follower list by placing them into specifically-named circles, such as Patients, Staff and New Prospects. The more circles you have, the more authority you will convey.

4. **Share Relevant Media:** When you share what's new, which is the Google+ Business version of the social media post, you will be able to share photos, links, videos or schedule events just by clicking the proper button. Remember that social media posts that contain media gather more conversions than non-media posts, more often than not.

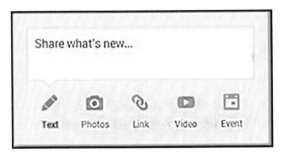

5. **Add Multiple Managers:** Just like Facebook, Google+ Business allows you to select multiple administrators, which it calls Managers, to help control the content and connect with other Google+ users and businesses. Take advantage of this ability by assigning posting abilities to your office staff.

6. **Start a Hangout:** Google+ Business makes it easy to host your very own webinar where you can hold your audience captive while you inform, educate and entertain. You might schedule a Hangout every thirty days to announce a Patient of the Month, whereby the

winner must be present in the Hangout to win. Talk about ramping up online attendance and social engagement!

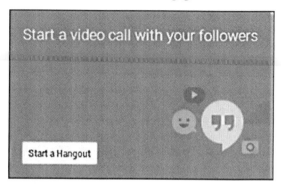

7. **Share What's New Often:** We recommend that you post on Google+ Business at least three times per week, but once per day is even better. While it is acceptable to share the same content you share on Facebook and Twitter, occasionally post new content to give people a reason to check out all three social networks.

***

Step 4: Create a YouTube Channel

In case you were not previously aware, Google owns the world's most popular video sharing site, YouTube. In fact, the search giant recently merged YouTube with its Google+ platform. Since you already created a Google+ account in the previous chapter, you already have a YouTube account by default. Click on www.YouTube.com and find the Home tab in the top left corner of your screen. Then select My Channel.

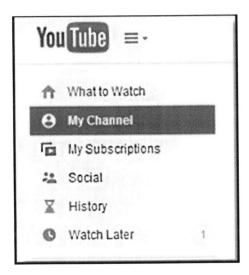

Your YouTube channel is where you will manage the videos you upload, as well as manage and communicate with your viewing audience. YouTube will encourage you to dress your channel up by offering several Channel tips.

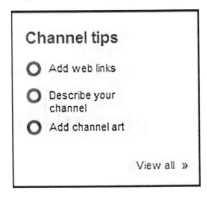

Take the advice YouTube offers by adding web links to your website pages, blogs and other social profiles. Describe your channel just as you did on your Facebook, Twitter and Google+ Business pages and add channel art, which is a photo that accurately represents your practice's channel and the message it hopes to convey.

How to Get the Most Out of Your YouTube Account

Here are seven tips to remember to get the most conversions out of your YouTube channel.

1. **Upload Targeted & Engaging Videos:** Do your best to create videos that your prospects and patients want to see. You may

show off a new piece of dental equipment in action, showcase your staff and their improved phone and customer service skills, highlight some of your VIPatients and their face-to-camera testimonials or you might even showcase some of your treatments and procedures in an intimate in-office exposé. Find out what your audience is most interested in and deliver that content in the form of ready-to-view-and-post YouTube videos.

2. **Publish & Share Your Videos Often:** We recommend that you publish a new video to YouTube at least once per week. Then share those videos on your web pages, blogs and social networks.

3. **Include Your Keywords:** Come up with any terms that you think people will type into the YouTube search box or the Google search box to find your practice and use those very terms in your channel description, video titles and video descriptions to increase your chances of being found online.

4. **Flex Your Title Creation Skills:** Now that you are a professional at developing titles that bring readers in droves, extend that talent to your YouTube channel to create video titles that guarantee views and conversions.

5. **Attractive Video Descriptions:** Your descriptions should make people want to watch your videos. Make your videos seem exciting and give hints as to the content. For an added search engine boost, include your practice NAP (remember, that's your name, address and phone number) with every video description you publish.

6. **Proper Video Length:** Provided that you have done nothing else to improve engagement with your videos, the shorter your videos happen to be, the higher the view count is likely to go. For best results, keep your videos from 30 seconds to 2-minutes to appease and increase conversions with those viewers who possess the shortest of attention spans.

7. **Calls-to-Action:** Accompany your videos with CTA's like "If you liked this video, send us an email and tell us so." Or, "To see more videos that feature this amazing technology at work, visit our website at www.GenericDental.com/treatments/dental-technology/" where you can then list a series of videos on the same subject. Remember, if you want people to view, click, ring or visit, ask for what you want and you'll be more likely to receive it.

How to Upload a Video to YouTube

You may think that you need high-quality and overly-polished videos to succeed, much like the ones you see on TV. However, studies show that people respond to impromptu videos much more than they do overly-produced ones. Look at the reality TV phenomena. People crave reality on film and this actually works to your advantage.

This means that you don't need expensive video and editing equipment and you don't need to hire actors or script writers or a crafts-services company to feed all the actors and behind-the-scenes personnel for an entire day's shoot. Instead, you can use your smartphone, tablet or any video camera at all.

If you wish to edit your videos, YouTube has a built-in film editor you can use, background music you can download and there are many free video editors online. Yet as long as your videos are informative, educational and entertaining, you won't need much editing at all. Go for rawness and your audience will appreciate the fact that your message isn't overly marketed, as many brand videos are today.

When your videos are ready to go live, visit your YouTube dashboard and click the Upload button near the gear icon in the top right corner of your screen.

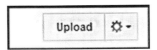

Give it a try and you will see that uploading and optimizing videos is so easy, it's almost addictive once you get the hang of it.

***

Step 5: Create Profiles on Pinterest, Instagram & Vine

It is advised that you stick with the top four social networks before you venture on to use any others, with three major exceptions.

Pinterest

Pinterest is a visually-focused social network. People go there strictly for the images and videos that others post or Pin, as the site calls it, to their virtual bulletin boards. You can sign in with your Facebook account and, once signed in, you can proceed to decorate your bulletin board any way you like.

It is recommended that you Pin staff and patient photos and videos to your board in all their high-definition brilliance.

Only implement Pinterest if you can keep up with your Pins, Re-Pins (which act like retweets) and communication with other Pinterest members.

These next two social networks are app-based, which means that they are better accessed on a smartphone or other mobile device, such as a tablet. You can search for and download the apps by visiting your device's respective app store.

Instagram

Owned by Facebook, this image-focused platform allows you to use your smartphone or mobile device to snap photos that can then be edited with various filters and focus options. Recently the platform added video capabilities. You are only allowed 15 seconds, so make your videos really good. Instagram photos and videos are perfect for showing posed and candid shots of your staff, practice and patients.

Vine

Owned by Twitter, Vine allows you to take six-second looping videos and publish them for the world to see. The site offers in-platform video editing and an easy upload process. Just point, shoot and publish.

Your Instagram and Vine creations can then be shared on your other social networks, such as Facebook, Twitter, Google+ Business and Pinterest.

Organizing & Managing Your Social Marketing Campaign

We recommend that you assign one or more people in your office to manage your social networks, as well as post and respond to messages as they come in. You might want to keep a binder in the office that tracks activity and that contains logins and passwords for the various social accounts we have mentioned.

Come up with a post quota that must be followed daily and reviewed weekly in order to maximize engagement and conversions. A schedule might include 1 Facebook post, 3 tweets, and 1 Google+ Business post per day. You might then schedule 1 video to be posted per week, either uploaded to YouTube or uploaded to Instagram or Vine. Mix it up for best results.

Be careful of falling into the trap of only hiring one person to manage all of your social media accounts. If that person is out sick or let go, your social accounts may suffer. Delegate responsibilities as necessary and test your results to determine post content and frequency by gauging the responses of your prospects and patients. Don't worry; we will soon show you how to examine and test your social marketing results in a coming section.

***

Spend some time getting used to the preceding social networks and the act of communicating with your audience. Once you feel that you are comfortable enough with this step to continue, you will be ready to move on to the next section of your dental Internet marketing campaign: Setting up your first email marketing campaign.

Chapter 7: Add Email Marketing to the Mix

Email marketing used to be the best way to target prospective patients until social media came along. That is why we included social media before this section. Normally, email marketing would come right after blog marketing, as an email subscriber opt-in form is the perfect complement to a website or blog.

When you entice prospects and patients to sign up to your permission-only subscriber list, you will gain a captive audience that you can then communicate with anytime you have something to say. With a targeted list, you can keep your subscribers in the loop anytime you add a new webpage or update an old one. You can blast out a message anytime you publish a new blog post or receive an intriguing comment on a previous post.

You can announce the creation of your social media accounts, build excitement over your new practice specials, discounts and free offers; you can announce patients of the month, new treatment service offerings, new technologies that will benefit your audience and, best of all, you can send personal messages to select-patients-only, such as sending out birthday, wedding anniversary and even first appointment anniversary celebrations.

Email marketing is cost-effective, easy to implement (as you will soon see) and it provides an opportunity to earn massively on your original investment. In fact, studies show that for every $1 that you invest in email marketing, you will receive an average of $44.25 back. Not bad for a dental Internet marketing technique that doesn't cost a thing to implement.

Keep in mind that while the email marketing platform that we are about to show you is indeed free, there are many paid options that offer improved reach and functionality. For our purposes, we are going to start you out on the free version of email marketing, which still gives you plenty of functionality to work with and one that will be perfect for your needs.

Step 1: Create a Self-Hosted Email Account

When you signed up for a Google+ account, you were provided with a Gmail address, which you may have been using up to this point to sign into your various online accounts. This is perfectly acceptable. Google is used by billions of people all over the world and Gmail is a very legitimate email source.

But if you want to lend even more legitimacy to your brand, you will want to use an email address that is connected to your domain name, such as doctorbruce@GenericDental.com. You may have been enticed to purchase an email account from your domain registrar at the time of checkout. If you opted out, you can set up your own dedicated email account on the web hosting service you chose in the beginning prior to setting up your website.

Since we used HostGator in our example of how to establish web host service, we will now show you how to set up a self-hosted email account using that very service. If you chose a different web host provider, refer to their documentation for how to set up a free self-hosted email account. You will likely find the process very similar to the steps listed below.

To create your new email account, visit your HostGator cPanel and click on the icon within the Mail section marked Email Accounts.

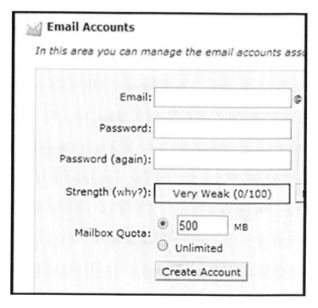

Here you will be able to create an unlimited amount of accounts. You will first be asked to select the title of your email address. Some examples include:

admin@GenericDental.com
webmaster@GenericDental.com
doctorbruce@GenericDental.com

Ensure that your email address is easy to remember so that prospects and patients will be more inclined to use it to send a message to your office. Select a difficult-to-guess password and that is all there is to it. You now have your very own office email address that can be used for all of your online accounts.

In fact, we recommend that you go through all of your accounts and proceed to their Settings sections to change the email address you originally provided to the new email address you have just created. This will keep all of your messages coming in to the same inbox, thus improving the odds that the messages will be seen and responded to.

Once you are finished creating your email address, you will notice that, in this same section, you can change your password, change the quota (though you can choose to receive an unlimited amount of emails) and delete your account at any time.

To access your account to read and send emails, select the More tab and choose Access Webmail.

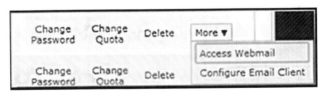

Here is a hint that you can use to keep your email addresses and messages organized. Download the free email management platform Thunderbird by Mozilla by visiting www.mozilla.org/thunderbird. Thunderbird will allow you to keep track of multiple emails from the same dashboard, ensuring that you always see and respond to emails the moment they come in.

***

Step 2: Create an Email Marketing Account

Email marketing becomes infinitely easier when you employ the help of an email marketing platform. You can think of these platforms much like social media platforms.

Like Facebook, Twitter or Google+, the various email marketing platforms on the market will allow you to manage your followers, otherwise known as subscribers, and communicate with those followers in all new ways, namely by sending targeted newsletters and emails.

While there are many paid email marketing platforms that offer a range of innovative products and services to accompany your account, we are going to begin with a free email marketing platform that is by no means a slouch. The platform is known as Mail Chimp, though there is also AWeber, GetResponse, Constant Contact and many others.

We advise that you start off with a free Mail Chimp account before you move on to paid services with more advanced functionality.

How to Sign Up with Mail Chimp

Mail Chimp offers free sign up and most of the platform's basic services to all of its users, as long as you stay within 2000 subscribers and 12,000 emails per month. You can always upgrade your account later on for $10 per month if you wish to accommodate more subscribers and receive unlimited access to more advanced functions and processes.

For our purposes, we advise you to stick with the free account, which can be accessed by visiting www.MailChimp.com and clicking the Sign Up Free button prominently displayed on the Home page.

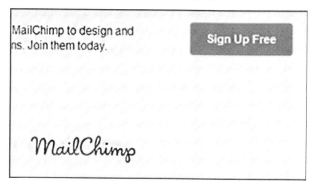

At this point the platform asks you to fill out some basic information, such as your email address, a username and a password. After that page, you will be asked more involved questions like your full name, the number of people in your organization, the age and name of your practice, your office address, domain name, industry type and time zone. You will also be asked to upload a profile photo.

Click Save and Get Started when you are finished with this section to be whisked away to your Mail Chimp Dashboard.

How to Navigate the Mail Chimp Dashboard

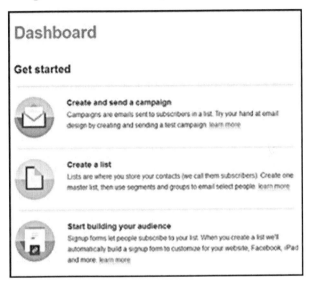

As you can see, Mail Chimp has made it very easy for beginners to become acclimated to their platform. The dashboard is separated into three primary sections:

- **Create and Send a Campaign:** This is where you will create your email messages and newsletters to send out to your audience.
- **Create a List:** In this section, you can import lists and manage all current lists with ease.
- **Start Building your Audience:** Here is where you will create your sign up forms to be placed on your website, blog and social media accounts.

There is also a side menu where you can manage your email marketing campaigns and lists, file reports, set up autoresponders (triggered messages that go out if prospects take specific actions) and a search function to find any campaign or contact information that you may find yourself looking for.

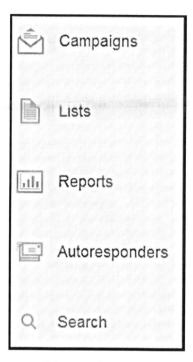

For now, you are interested in creating your first campaign. Choose the option that allows you to send an email to yourself for now and click submit to be taken to the Mail Chimp Campaign Builder, where you will be asked to list specific campaign details.

***

Step 3: Design Your First Email Marketing Campaign

Click on the Mail Chimp Campaign Builder to begin creating your first email marketing campaign that can be sent out to new patients, prospects, current patients and former patients alike.

How to Use the Mail Chimp Campaign Builder

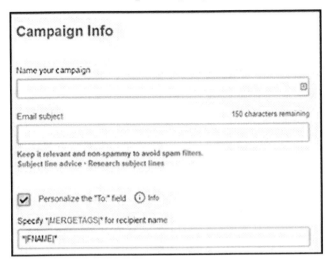

Your Email Campaign Name

The name of your campaign is for internal use only. It is a name for you to classify and organize your campaigns and will only be seen by you. Choose something memorable, such as GenericDental Campaign #1.

From Name and Address

The From Name and From email address will show up in your subscribers' inboxes next to your subject line. These should be instantly recognizable as belonging to your practice for best results. Use the advice above for creating a self-hosted email account that includes your domain name to lend your email messages extra credibility.

Email Subject Line

Out of all of the elements that comprise the typical email, the subject line is by far the most important. A potential reader will look at your subject line and decide within seconds whether or not to open your email. Today's email subscribers don't want to be lied to and they don't like to be tricked. Screaming at them in all caps that their teeth will fall out if they don't open your emails with five or six exclamation points following your subject line is not the way to go. Don't annoy your subscribers; entice them!

Your subject lines should be short, targeted and should give some hint as to the contents of the email in question. In other words, what will the reader get out of opening your email? If you can convey the basic idea and tease without giving away the whole enchilada, you will receive far more open rates and, potentially, conversions.

In email marketing, a conversion is said to happen when a reader opens the email and when action is taken, such as when a link to your website is clicked, a video is watched or a phone number is called.

To help you receive more open rates, we urge you to use Mail Chimp's new Email Subject Line Researcher Project. The project will check your subject lines against millions of others to provide you with the highest probability of opens and conversions. While this tool can help you hone your subject line creation skills, only data gleaned from your audience is the true litmus test of success. Later, we will show you how to test and tweak your email marketing messages for even greater effect.

Personalization

Next, Mail Chimp will ask you if you wish to personalize your messages for each recipient; and we recommend that you do, in fact, include personalization with every message you send. This will enable you to list the person's first name in the subject line, for example, which will increase the chances of the person opening and responding to the message in question.

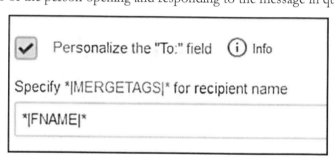

When you set personalization, you will be able to click on the tab marked 'Merge tag cheatsheet' anytime you are writing a new message.

With a list of Merge Tags, you will have multiple means of personalization at your disposal - as long as you are thorough at collecting personal information from your prospects and patients - as well as various quick and easy ways to embed social media links into the bodies of the email messages themselves.

Experiment with this personalization process to empower all of your future emails and, most of all, to gauge the response rates of your audience.

Near the bottom of this screen is a Tracking tab, which will allow you to track your conversions.

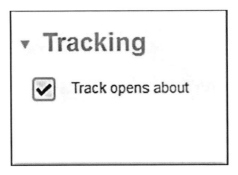

For our purposes, we are going to stay with the default options selected and proceed to the next tab down the page: The Social Media tab.

The Social Media tab allows you to link your Mail Chimp to your Facebook and Twitter accounts; and you are encouraged to do so. This makes it easy for your recipients to share your newsletters and emails with their social friends and followers, potentially bringing more email subscribers your way.

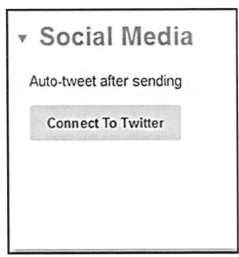

Under More Options, select both options that read Auto-convert video so that you can share your latest video marketing offerings and the one that opts to keep your emails out of your recipients' spam folders.

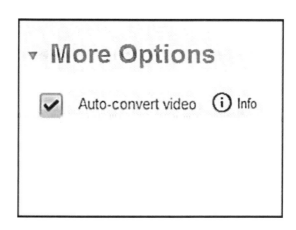

Keep in mind that you can change the above information anytime you send a new message to your audience. The above will set these options as your default settings so that you don't have to reset them every time you get ready to send a new message to one or more people

When you are ready to send your first message, click Next and proceed to the Email Campaign Designer.

How to Design Your Email Marketing Messages

Mail Chimp provides you with quite a few options for designing any type of newsletter or email you can think up. You can select the email designer, for instance, which allows you to create templates from scratch. This is ideal if you have a set design in mind and the expertise to maximize your results.

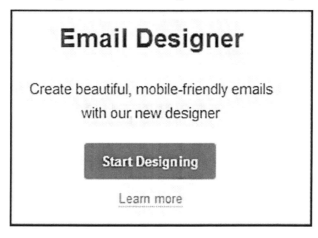

We recommend that you begin your foray into email marketing by thinking minimally. Choose the classic templates or the icon that is marked Predesigned templates.

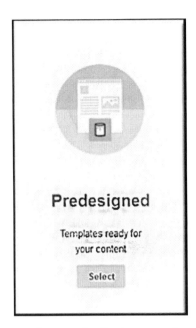

Predesigned

Templates ready for
your content

Select

Browse through the templates and edit the ones that catch your eye to fit your needs. Remember to use your office colors, fonts that are easy to read and to implement images, video and other media when appropriate.

Plain Text Emails

The above options are for sending HTML newsletters and emails. HTML (short for Hypertext Markup Language) is a type of computer code that allows your recipients to see your overall template design, including all colors, images, video and other media, as well as your links, logo and social media buttons.

Some recipients may opt to view your emails in plain text, which will show your email in just that, plain text, without all the bells and whistles. This may be due to security reasons, as HTML emails are sometimes used by hackers to spread nasty viruses. Some browsers for the hearing impaired also use text emails to read the messages aloud. These browser programs cannot see your emails, so you should do your best to provide readable content whenever possible. Plain text emails solve this problem beautifully. We recommend that you send both HTML and plain text to every recipient for best results.

Mail Chimp gives you a chance to preview and edit your email in plain text to ensure that your email translates perfectly, even though none of your media will actually appear on the recipients' end. Spend a second reading through your email and correcting mistakes before you proceed to the next step.

***

Step 4: Confirm & Send Your First Email

Mail Chimp allows you to revise your list, subject line, reply email address, tracking options, HTML email and plain text email designs, as well as your email authentication options before you hit Send. Check to make sure everything is perfect, because once you hit send you have fully committed; and there are certainly no backsies in email marketing.

***

Step 5: Comprise & Organize Your Subscriber List

Before you send your first message, you will need to create your first email subscriber list. Right now you don't have any subscribers, so when you try to send your first message, Mail Chimp will notify you that there is a problem that needs your attention. Click the Resolve button to create your subscriber list.

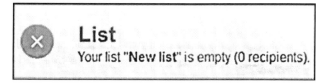

Keep in mind that you can also travel back to your Mail Chimp dashboard to click the Lists option on the menu on the left hand side to access your lists at any time.

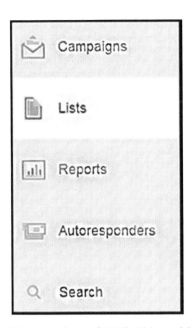

Once you are in the Lists section of Mail Chimp, hit the button marked Create List in the top right corner of your screen. Here is where you can add subscribers manually or import entire lists from a variety of sources.

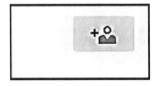

Keep in mind that for your email marketing campaign to receive the highest amounts of conversions, you will want to keep your subscriber list permission-based. The best way to get subscribers to opt-in to receive your messages is to place a sign up form on your website, blog and social media accounts.

The moment subscribers opt-in and leave their personal information, Mail Chimp will autorespond with a confirmation email, ensuring that your subscribers give their explicit permission to receive your email marketing messages.

It is important never to abuse your privileges once you have been given access to a recipients' inboxes. We recommend accompanying your opt-in sign up forms with a message informing your subscribers that you will never sell, trade, give away or abuse their contact information once it is in your possession.

When you are ready to compile your first Internet marketing list, proceed to the tab marked Sign up forms within the New List section.

How to Design a Mail Chimp Sign Up Form

A sign up form is a text box that asks prospects to enter a specified amount of information, such as a name and email address. Just as Mail Chimp gives you several tools for designing the appearance of your emails, you receive the same functionality for designing your sign up forms.

We recommend selecting the option marked Form Integrations, which will allow you to create sign up forms for platforms like Twitter and WordPress.

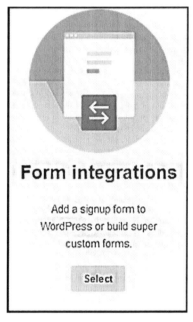

Here you can link your email subscription list to your Twitter account, enabling you to extend your reach and grow your list organically with every tweet you send.

We also want you to click on the Learn More button under the WordPress integration option.

This will bring you to a page where you can download the Mail Chimp WordPress Plugin.

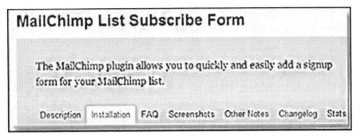

MailChimp List Subscribe Form

The MailChimp plugin allows you to quickly and easily add a signup form for your MailChimp list.

Description | Installation | FAQ | Screenshots | Other Notes | Changelog | Stats

Just as you downloaded the All in One SEO plugin earlier, download and unzip the Mail Chimp plugin the same way. You will then be able to seamlessly merge your sign up forms with your website and blog.

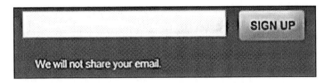

SIGN UP

We will not share your email.

How to Write Engaging Newsletters & Emails

If you want every one of your marketing emails to hit their mark, put these ten email writing best practices to good use.

1. **Get to the Point Quickly:** People reading their emails don't have time to read pages-and-pages of anything. Stick to around 200 words and use short sentences and paragraphs to keep readers paying attention.

2. **Talk One-on-One:** When writing your emails, it helps to form a composite of the ideal subscriber in your mind; then write your messages to that person. Write to this person as if you were in the same room speaking with him/her in your lobby using a professional and lighthearted tone.

3. **Links & Media:** Your newsletters and emails will be seen as offering more value if you include links wherever appropriate, such as when you are referencing a website, blog or video. You should have already accumulated a series of high-quality images and videos from your website, blog and social media marketing efforts. Here is your chance to keep sharing that content with all of your email marketing subscribers.

4. **Be Straight Forward:** Never lie to your subscribers or promise things that you can't, won't or don't follow through on. Your audience must come to trust you and see you as the dominant leader

in your field. If you lose their trust even a little bit, you will have a very difficult time getting it back.

5. **Use Preview Panes:** Mail Chimp allows you to include a bit of text that will show up on mobile browsers before the message is fully opened. Use this box to its maximum advantage to further entice your recipients to open and read.

   Use calls-to-action and announce the benefits of your email messages in your preview panes for best results. For example, one of your preview panes might read, "Open now to receive $50 off new patient exams!"

6. **Break-Up Content:** Just as you do with web and blog writing, break up your email content with short, concise paragraphs, bolded subheaders and bullet points wherever appropriate.

7. **Offer Value:** Every email you send should inform, educate, entertain or offer. Give your subscribers a reason to open the messages you send.

8. **Urgent Calls-to-Action:** Let your recipients know what you want them to do with strong calls-to-action like Call Now, Click Here and Watch This Video.

9. **Proper Email Scheduling:** We recommend that you send an informative newsletter once per month to all recipients that includes improvements to your practice, as well as news and information about the practice and the industry as a whole. Then send out supplemental emails that promote new blog posts, video uploads and special offers. The more emails you send, the longer you will remain on the minds of your subscribers. To find a schedule your audience responds to, you might want to conduct a poll with your audience to find out how often they wish to receive your messages.

10. **Segment Your List:** Mail Chimp allows you to segment your main subscriber list for the purposes of sending highly-targeted messages to the proper recipients. You might have a segment labeled prospects, one labeled patients and one labeled former patients. You can then send a welcome message to your prospects, an appointment reminder to your current patients and a third message that can go out to your former patients to entice them to

return. Use segmentation whenever possible to further improve your email marketing results.

***

Step 6: Write Your First Public Email Marketing Message

You can craft or edit your email messages at any time during the Campaign Builder process by selecting the term *Design* in the breadcrumbs bar near the bottom of the page.

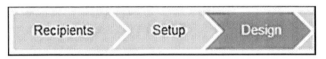

After you select your template, you will be able to edit your message, which you will notice is very similar to the way you create and edit posts and pages in WordPress.

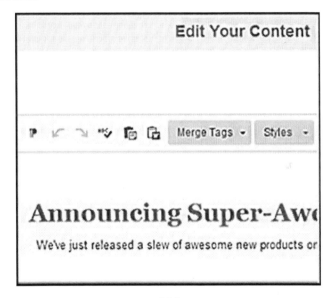

***

Write your newsletters and emails and send them often. If you are ever stuck on what to write about, here are three email marketing templates to help you get started.

3 Email Templates for Dental Practices

To help your messages succeed and stand out in any recipient's inbox, here are a few email templates you can use for your own purposes. Read them over, go over them with your staff and alter them to suit your own practice needs.

New Prospects

Since new prospects may not yet be familiar with your practice, you must remind your prospects why you are contacting them. At the same time, let them know that they were noticed by your practice staff and that you are looking forward to meeting them in person. Finally, give them a reason to read and respond.

Subject: [First Name], thank you for calling our office. Special offer inside.

Hello **[First Name]**,

Thank you for calling GenericDental. Your phone call managed to brighten up the entire office. I hope we succeeded in answering all of your questions. If you still have questions or if you would like to schedule an appointment, we just might have an opening that is perfect for you. Call us right now at 555-1395.

Act now and receive $50 off your first oral exam. I hope to see you in our office very soon.

Regards,

Bobbie Sue Riley
Office Administrator
Generic Dental

Tips for Sending Emails to New Prospects

1. There is no need to mention your practice name in the subject line. Your From line and email address should tell your subscribers all they need to know about where the message originated.
2. Make your messages short and rewarding.
3. Use personalization to make prospects feel unique and special.

***

Current Patients

Reward your current patients for being subscribers and push referrals whenever you can.

Subject: [First Name], watch this video for a good laugh.

Hello **[First Name]**,

I just saw this video and thought of you. Remember during your last exam when Dr. Nunzio told you to brush and floss regularly? This is what happens when you don't do either of those things.

[Embedded Video]

But seriously, thank you for being a valued patient. I wanted to give you a coupon for $100 off Teeth Whitening. Just click here to print your coupon. Also, if you recommend us to someone else, we'll give you an extra $100 off.

I can't wait to see you at your next appointment.

Regards,

Bobbie Sue Riley
Office Administrator
Generic Dental

Tips for Sending Emails to Current Patients

1. Always deliver the very best quality to remain in your patients' good graces and to entice referrals.
2. Leave links and media to improve the value that your emails offer.
3. Use common language and humor to increase the odds that your emails will be forwarded and shared.

***

Former Patients

Let former patients know exactly why you are contacting them and give them a reason to read and respond.

Subject: [First Name], here is a special offer from GenericDental just for you!

Hello **[First Name]**,

We've missed you in the office lately. How long has it been now? I wanted to let you know that so much has happened since we've last seen you. We upgraded our waiting room, added new dentist chairs and we even have tablets you can use to watch movies while we examine, clean and treat your smile.

We'd love to help you become our patient again. To help you in your decision to return, we wanted to offer you a free exam and teeth cleaning. Act now to take advantage of this offer by calling me right now at 555-1395.

Regards,

Bobbie Sue Riley
Office Administrator
Generic Dental

Tips for Sending Emails to Former Patients

1. Let former patients know exactly what they've been missing.
2. Mention upgrades, specials and free offers to entice former patients to return.
3. Provide an urgent call-to-action to improve conversions.

***

Just like Mint Dental when they reached this stage, your dental Internet marketing campaign is beginning to come together nicely; and the only money you've spent so far was the measly amount you spent to secure your domain name and web hosting account.

You can experience a lot of results with these free and low-cost methods, and Mint Dental did just that. But if you want the phone to ring more often and for the office lobby to remain full, it would be wise to venture into more advanced forms of dental Internet marketing. That is where your path now leads. After you are familiar with the processes listed in the preceding chapters, turn the page and let's get started.

Part 3: Advanced Dental Internet Marketing
- Going Deeper

Mint Dental Develops a Paid Internet Marketing Campaign

With his practice's website in place, a functioning blog, active social media accounts, a regular newsletter and strategically sent email marketing messages, Mint Dental found itself steadily climbing the local market ladder. But being the ambitious professional he is, Dr. M. still wasn't completely satisfied. He wanted more.

That's when we decided to take Mint Dental deeper into the world of Dental Internet marketing. We conducted extensive keyword research and established a paid Internet advertising campaign that put the doctor's ads in front of relevant search engine users online.

This is when we introduced the doctor and his practice to the more advanced methods of search engine optimization. The following steps will provide you with a deeper meaning of how the search engines operate and how you can use that knowledge to drive even more conversions, leads and high-quality patients to your practice.

These are the steps that helped Mint Dental become the $5 million practice in a single year, and they will help you, too. First, we feel it is important to educate you on the proper methods of search engine optimization and how they can be used to help your online presence truly connect with - and attract - your growing audience.

Chapter 8: An Introduction to Search Engine Optimization (SEO)

Up until this point we have taught you how to put a basic web presence in place. To make your web presence even more powerful and to ensure that anyone using a computer, smartphone or other mobile device can find your practice information wherever they happen to be, we are now going to teach you all about the search engines and the practice known as search engine optimization or SEO.

The Science Behind the Search Engines

The search engines are nothing more than automated programs that seek to organize the web and all of its content for one single purpose: to help you find what you need. Yes, you. Google cares about you and all the others who use the platform; and its job is to sift through the countless websites, blogs, social media accounts and other content – with more being added every day – in order to deliver the most valuable and relevant search results as they relate to your original search query.

In order to deliver the most accurate results, Google and the other search engines use powerful algorithms, which are mathematical equations that are constantly being tweaked, upgraded and improved upon in order to accommodate the constant influx of websites, images, videos, infographics, sound files, etc. etc. ad infinitum that show up online.

Search engines have existed in some form or another since the nineties. Back then sites were ranked primarily by the content on their pages. In other words, keywords were the prime order of the day; and it was common for webmasters to congregate in online chat rooms to discuss how to rank their websites prominently in the search engines on online forums and bulletin boards.

Then Google arrived on the scene at the turn of the century and introduced the world to Page Rank, which sought to categorize websites depending on their content and their levels of authority within their given niches or categories. The higher the Page Rank number, the more prominently that site's pages would rank in the search results.

Page Rank was also able to be passed from authority sites to lesser known sites by way of linking; thus giving those unpopular sites a boost in the Search Engine Results Pages or SERPs.

It didn't take long for webmasters to catch on to how the Page Rank system worked and some webmasters tried to game the system in an effort to dominate the SERPs for the keywords they were optimizing for. They began to stuff their pages with keywords and gather links from authoritative sites by the dozens, hundreds and even thousands in a desperate attempt to dominate the search results, even if those authority sites had nothing to do with the original site in question.

While this gaming of the system helped the webmasters shoot to the top of the SERPs and many of them made tons of money hand over fist, the results of this cheating of the search results infuriated Google.

Not only were these webmasters manipulating a system that was put in place to help search users better navigate the web, but the websites that were at the heart of the scandal were hardly viewed as being of the best quality, even at the time; and not by a long shot.

In fact, most of these sites were nothing more than blank pages stuffed with one or two keywords repeated over and over. This is hardly what Google had in mind when it sought to categorize and deliver excellent content to the masses.

The fact that most of these cheating websites were of a lower quality was not surprising. Most webmasters looking to game the system were looking for the shortcut to riches; and providing eye-catching web design, interesting and entertaining web copy and all the other elements that go into providing a memorable web experience just wasn't something these guys - and gals - were willing to do.

Google sought to stifle this hijacking of the SERPs by altering its algorithm. The moment this happened, all of those sites that were enjoying inflated rankings plummeted in the search results. Money was lost, businesses were ruined and more than a few angry webmasters vented their frustrations about Google everywhere they could, usually in the most popular Internet forums of the day. And so the Dance began.

SEO historians liken the race to game Google's system as a dance for a very good reason. Google will come out with an algorithm change that is designed to thwart any cheating and unscrupulous webmasters will inevitably study those changes to develop innovative ways to beat it, and so this dance has continued almost since the beginning of Google's reign at the top of the search engine hierarchy.

Around 2003, Google stopped resisting and started helping. For the first time, the search giant offered tips and suggestions for attaining the top positions for relevant keyword terms. And Google has done so ever since with Webmaster Tools, the section of Google that provides tutorials and advice to webmasters. We will discuss and use Webmaster Tools in an upcoming section.

During that time, Google taught webmasters how to research the best keywords to make it easy for search users to find them on the web; how to attain backlinks, those links that lead from other sites to your site; and to attain relevancy through online relationships.

Over the years, Google has taken into account all of the newly existing technologies and user trends in order to deliver the highest quality results. For instance, in 2010, Google announced that it was using social signals in its search results, which is an indication that your target audience is sharing your web content on social media.

And yet the search giant has struggled to fight against what are known today as black hat SEO tactics, those methods that are used to game its system, and has consistently altered its algorithm ever since. There is never a warning when a new algorithm occurs and no one really knows how each one works. Google will sometimes release snippets of information to webmasters, but much of the change that happens is considered very top secret. This undercover tweaking process usually stops the cheating; at least for a while, until some other crafty individuals come up with new tactics to boost rankings without actually having to work for it.

People try all sorts of ways to cheat Google, such as keyword stuffing, which we mentioned, buying thousands of backlinks, buying social media connections and by scraping content; a process where your content is copied and then slapped onto a lower-quality site in order to attain higher rankings.

Google is watching for all of these tactics and they are only mentioned because you are urged not to use them. Follow the techniques in this book and explore Webmaster Tools to absorb Google's instructions for using its search engine for maximum benefit. If you go for gradual and consistent results and you use the proper amounts of keywords, build your links slowly and organically over time and you simply try to provide the best experience to your visitors that you possibly can, you can only assume that Google will reward you.

Google Updates and the Resulting Aftermaths

Every time there is a new Google update, there is constant online chatter where you have people claiming that Google destroyed their business or even their lives. You can almost always bet that these people have succumbed to the temptation of using black hat tactics for the promise of immediate and substantial gains. When it comes to SEO, what comes fast can quickly fall and businesses that try to cheat Google usually do fall immediately following a new algorithm update.

Sites that use white hat SEO tactics, on the other hand, typically see no change or very slight changes when a new algorithm update happens. This is due to the fact that the sites in question are doing exactly what they are supposed to be doing: helping their visitors become more educated, informed and entertained.

Through the years, Google's updates have taken on many monikers, most recently names like Panda, Penguin and Hummingbird. And each one comes with a different set of parameters that webmasters must keep in mind.

Despite all the changes, the way Google indexes its search results goes a little something like this. Automated bots are regularly sent out to scan or crawl all of the content that can be found online. These bots will analyze your website, the colors you use, the speed with which your site loads, the content you provide, the keyword terms you have used most frequently and whether people have shared your website and its content on social media.

Your site information will then be indexed for use in future relevant search results. Google uses over 200 factors to help determine the quality and relevancy of a particular web page for the purposes of accurate ranking. If you can maximize colors, content, site speed and all the other elements Google and other search engine bots might check for, you just might reach the pinnacle of your field in the SERPs.

We have already provided you with a number of white hat SEO tactics for ranking prominently in Google, but this chapter is going to go a bit further. Instead of going through the immense Webmaster Tools library, we are going to do our best to break down the process of SEO in an easily-digestible manner for you right now.

The steps you are about to learn come straight from Google and are considered legitimate, scrupulous and the proper way to stay in Google's good graces. To begin, we are going to start by breaking down the typical search results page.

***

The Anatomy of Search Engine Results Pages (SERPs)

To view the SERPs in action, search for a keyword, such as "Dentist in Altus Oklahoma" and see what Google comes up with.

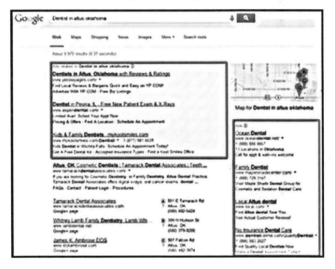

When the page comes up, you will notice that there are two types of listings: paid listings and natural or organic listings. The organic listings are the ones we have focused on up until this point. By including the proper amounts of keywords, ensuring relevant and quality backlinks and by focusing on providing a valuable web experience to your audience, it is your hope that your website and all of its related pages will show up in the first few spots on the very first page of the Google SERPs.

If you don't want to go through the trouble of optimizing your website organically, there is always paid online advertising.

Since Google search happens to be a free service, you may wonder how the search giant makes its money. Allow us to introduce you to the Google Adwords paid online advertising platform, which is where Google makes most of its money by the truckload.

You can get a jump start on landing on the first page of Google and all the benefits that come from such an honor if you have enough money to pay for it. We will cover paid online advertising in greater detail in an upcoming chapter, but for right now understand that advertisers stock their accounts with enough money to bid for top spots when searchers use relevant keyword terms to find what they are looking for. With the right ads and the right ad budget, you can put your dental services in front of decision makers who then have a high chance of becoming leads.

Ideally, you will want to reach the top spot of Google both organically and through paid advertising, thus doubling, tripling and even quadrupling your results.

For right now, focus on ranking organically with your already-constructed and launched basic Internet marketing web presence.

How Google Ranks Dentists

Keywords: Google will search through your site to determine which words or terms are repeated most often and will rank your site accordingly. This is why you will want to use specific keywords throughout your content on each page, most importantly the ones that have to do with your business, location and specialization.

Relevancy: Google has to determine which sites are the most relevant to users' search terms. Using the proper keywords in strategic locations on any given page can help immensely in this regard.

Legitimacy: Google has the tough job of determining if your site is an actual, valuable offering to your audience or if it is merely a site that has been thrown together for the purposes of scamming people. You can help Google in its decision by providing excellent graphics, content and useful information.

Authority: Google must be able to postulate that your website is the most valuable in your industry. In other words, are you providing more valuable and useful information than your competitors? If so, you will likely enjoy more prominent rankings than every dental professional in your general area.

Fresh Content: Google typically rewards fresh content with higher rankings than they do content that has remained the same for weeks, months or even years. To achieve more prominent rankings, you should produce new web content whenever possible. A blog updated every week or multiple times weekly might just give you the edge you need.

Public Perception: New studies show that most people view online reviews as being just as reputable as personal recommendations from friends and family. And many consumers today like to connect with their favorite brands and businesses on social media. Use this knowledge to your advantage by compiling profiles on sites like Facebook, Twitter, Yahoo, Yelp, Google+ Business, Yahoo Places and Insider Pages.

With this knowledge under your belt, we are going to help you rank prominently in Google and any other search engines that people may use to find your practice. We are going to begin where Google began over ten years ago, by examining the keywords your practice uses to entice prospects to become patients.

***

Keywords – the Foundation of Internet Marketing

Though Google and the other search engines are wary of keyword stuffing, they still rely heavily on keywords to help them decide where and how to rank a website in the SERPs. If you think about it, it's a pretty smart way of determining what a website is about. Take your dental website, for example. Google will employ the use of automated bots or spiders to crawl your website looking for any information it can use to determine its subject matter and level of quality. The bots are looking for keywords first and foremost.

Let's say that a Google user types 'dentist in Anchorage' into the search box and that you are, in fact, a dentist in Anchorage. If your website mentions the keywords, 'dentist in anchorage', you could potentially show up on the first spot on the first page of the search results. Cha-ching!

That is why it is very important that your website and all other web elements utilize the most important keywords of your industry so that you can rank prominently and receive all the traffic that comes from a top SERP position.

You can't just throw the keywords onto your pages, however, and you certainly can't keyword stuff like those black hat SEOers. There is an art form to keyword research and placement. Let's examine that art form now.

Short Tail vs. Long-tail Keywords

There are essentially two types of keywords – short tail and long-tail keywords. Short tail keywords represent one to three words and are very limited in scope. Then there are the long-tail keywords that typically consist of three or more words and are much more specific.

Short tail keywords are usually generic terms that are not very helpful in optimizing your sites for the search engines. Consider the effort Google has to put forth to yield relevant results for the short tail keyword "Dentist". Even the keyword "Dentist Office" is non-helpful. If you were to optimize for those terms, you would find your practice up against millions upon millions of other competitors who also use those terms in their web copy.

Today search users know to be much more specific if they are looking for a dentist's office, or any other person, place or thing they may be searching for. To find a dental practice today, users will most likely specify the location, the services they are shopping for, and other identifiers, such as their preferred insurance, to help narrow the search even more.

That is why it is much better to use long-tail keywords when optimizing for the search engines. A good long-tail keyword search term might be "Teeth whitening in Anchorage AK". See how specific that is? Google should have no trouble returning the listings of a few offices that specialize in teeth whitening in the Anchorage area.

Another good long-tail keyword term might be, "Emergency dentist Aetna insurance Dallas Tx". This tells Google to return emergency dentistry offices in Dallas that accept Aetna insurance.

The lesson here is to stay away from short tail keywords and to use more long-tail keywords in your website copy and throughout your other dental Internet marketing campaigns. No one is typing "Orthodontist" into Google, for instance. That single term is going to yield millions of websites from all over the world. Instead, people might type, "Orthodontist in Austin" or, "Orthodontist Invisalign Austin, Tx".

As a dental professional, you need to focus on the three primary types of keywords for dentists.

Three Keyword Types for Dentists

Our Internet marketing team focuses on dental practices specifically and in our experience there are three primary keywords for dentists.

1. **Services:** These are the terms that describe what you do you can help prospects and patients. They are your ver.. canals, cavities and wisdom teeth extraction keywords.

2. **Insurance Coverage:** Prospects considering your practice want to know that their insurance will be accepted and that they won't have too many out-of-pocket expenses. Your insurance keywords – Aetna, Blue Cross/Blue Shield, Medicaid and Humana – will drastically improve the quality of your leads.

3. **Geographical Area:** These are the state, city and suburb names - and zip code - that represent your practice area. As a dental professional, you rely heavily on local customers; and including geo-based keywords is the perfect way to bring more of your neighbors through your office door.

Use one type of keyword, a combination of two of the above or all three keyword types for best results.

Your job, as someone who is attempting to optimize your website, blog and social media accounts for the search engines, is to find the most searched-for long-tail keyword terms that also offer the least amount of competition. In this case, competition means webmasters like yourself who may be optimizing for the same terms.

Later, we have dedicated an entire section to keyword research and organization. For right now, we are going to teach you a few tricks of the trade for finding the most sought-after keywords so that you can give your basic web presence the edge it needs.

Basic Keyword Generation

Gather your dental team together for a brain-storming session and see how many keyword terms your group can come up with in a single session. Invite anyone to give their two cents and don't discard any ideas. It is best to keep the keywords that are mentioned during this exercise in a separate tab in your spreadsheet for easy organization and use later.

Remember to include your services, insurance coverage and geographical area as much as possible and to make the keywords long-tail by design. Google's most recent algorithm updates have begun to take into account every word that users might type into a search box.

This means that Google may be looking for entire sentences, such as "Dentist in New York that takes Aetna" or "Teeth whitening clinic in Austin that uses lasers". Your job is to write down as many terms as you can think of that Google users might type into the search box to find your practice. Google also takes into account synonyms and related terms, such as Titanium Post for Dental Implants, for example. Use this information to comprise your keyword list.

Here is another example. If your practice is a cosmetic dentistry service in White Plains, NY, your list might look like this.

White Plains cosmetic dentist NY 10601
White Plains NY smile makeover
Veneers in White Plains NY
Dental bridges White Plains New York Humana insurance

Once you have compiled your list, open your favorite browser to the Google homepage and search for your keywords in quotes. So for our first example, you will search for "white plains cosmetic dentist NY 10601". It may take some time to search for every keyword on your list, depending on how extensive your list happens to be, but doing so can give you important information that you can use to further improve all of your Internet marketing campaign efforts.

Searching in quotes tells Google to yield only those results where that particular keyword exists somewhere on the page and in that exact order. Without quotes, Google might return pages that only contain the words White Plains or that only contain Cosmetic Dentist. With quotes, you can be sure that Google is searching for the exact keyword term that you wish to examine and nothing else.

When the search results come up, spend some time clicking on the first few organic links that appear on the SERP. These are your primary competitors and the ones that you will be vying for search engine dominance over. By searching for your keyword terms this way, you can determine how popular the keywords are and how much competition there is for each one.

As an added tip, scroll to the bottom of the page and see if Google tries to suggest any keywords. The keywords at the bottom are typically the most searched-for keywords as they relate to the term you just entered. The terms that Google proposes can help you further hone your long-tail keyword list.

This is known as preliminary keyword research. If you want to continue your research to find the most searched-for and least competing keywords for your practice and services, here are a number of free and low-cost tools that you can use for that very purpose.

Keyword Research Tools

Google Trends

(www.google.com/trends)

This free tool from Google will allow you to enter your keywords to determine how they have ranked in the search engine from past to present. You can also view related keyword searches and regional activity, as well as a few other important details. This tool is great for narrowing down your keyword list.

5 Minute Site Tool

(http://5minutesite.com/local_keywords.php)

This free tool allows you to compile a list of local zip codes and neighborhood names. This tool is ideal for gathering the proper geographical keywords for your dental practice.

SpyFu

(www.spyfu.com)

This tool costs money, but there is a free trial. Designed for pay-per-click (PPC) paid advertising campaigns, SpyFu can tell you what keywords your competitors are ranking for and which ones are the most viable for search and PPC dominance.

SEO Tool Set

(www.seotoolset.com/tools/free_tools.html)

With both free and paid options, the SEO tool set allows you to enter up to twelve keywords at a time to see how they rank and how viable they are for your dental Internet marketing campaigns.

Google Adwords Keyword Planner

Considered the mac daddy of keyword tools, Google's proprietary keyword research client is reserved for Adwords customers only, which if you recall is Google's paid online advertising platform. We have included a full breakdown of the tool in a later section. For right now, use the tools above and proceed to the next section.

***

On-Site (On-Page) SEO – Optimizing Your Web Presence

When search engines like Google crawl your site looking for valuable and relevant information for the purposes of categorization and ranking, they typically do so from the top down. That is how we will approach this next section. Starting from the very top of your site – known as the header - all the way down to the bottom of your site – otherwise known as the footer – we are going to teach you how to optimize your site internally. This process is known as on-site or on-page SEO.

Metadata

Back before content management systems like WordPress existed, websites would have to be coded largely by hand. In order to provide valuable information to your audience and appease the search engines simultaneously, you would have had to have extensive knowledge of coding so that you entered the proper metadata behind the design, text and media that people could actually experience, read and see.

Metadata consists of internal code that is designed specifically to be read and processed by search engine bots, spiders or crawlers (These bots have different names depending on the search engine you are referencing). Thanks to WordPress and the All in One Plugin that we installed earlier in this book, entering your metadata is as easy as typing it onto the page.

Title & Description Tags

The first pieces of crucial metadata that search engines will read consists of Title and Description tags. Incidentally, these are the titles and descriptions that you read when you conduct a search engine query.

Conduct a Google search and examine the first organic link that shows up on the SERP. The title is the part you see in blue and the description is right underneath it.

Dental Implants | Mint Dental
www.mintdentalalaska.com/our-services/dental-implants ▾
★★★★★ Rating: 5 - 24 reviews
Mint Dental offers cosmetic dentistry services which includes dental Implants. We use the latest technology, contact ... Toll Free: 1-855-646-6468. Anchorage, AK.
More by Jon McNeil - in 36 Google+ circles

By manipulating the metadata within your website, you can actually determine what Google shows to prospects and patients when they conduct a relevant search.

You will want to write title and description tags for every page on your website. Again, thanks to WordPress and All in One, doing this is easy-peasy.

First, select Pages on the left hand pane of your WordPress dashboard. Then, select Add New. Or, if you want to write the metadata for one of your existing pages, select Pages and then find a page you have already created. Then select Edit underneath the page's title.

This will bring you to the WordPress page creation or edit screen. If you scroll down past the main content box, you will notice an All in One section. Here is where you will enter your title and description tags, as well as the keywords that you wish to be ranked for.

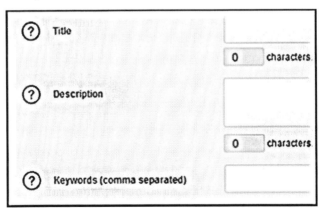

This information will give Google and the other search engines a heads up on where and how to rank this particular page.

How to Optimize Title and Description Tags

Earlier we recommended setting up your website's URL structure in a specific way. We also mentioned that you should keep this structure in a spreadsheet file. This same spreadsheet file can help you write and organize your title and description tags.

Your page title tags should include the name of your practice and at least one of your primary keywords. For best results, we recommend inserting geographic keywords in every title on every page. Shoot for under 70 characters for best results. To check your character count, do a Google search for a free letter/character counter and enter your title tags to check their validity.

GenericDental | Premium Dentistry in Austin | Most Insurance Accepted

Your description tags should include information about your practice and entice search users to click on your link or call your practice. For best results, include your phone number or other contact information. These should be 200 characters or less.

Visit GenericDental today and experience premium dentistry in a calm and soothing environment. Call today: 444-0111.

While it is important to use your keywords in your title tags, it's not as necessary to use them in your descriptions, but every bit helps. Just make sure that your titles and descriptions are accurate, legible and that every single one is unique for every page or post you publish. The search engines hate duplicate content and you will be penalized for copying content, especially in Google.

Media Tags

The next meta tags that are crucial to your website's optimization consist of image and video tags (and tags for all other types of media). Keep in mind that the search engines aren't just interested in the text on your website's individual pages. They are also interested in the images, photos, videos and sound bites. And luckily, WordPress makes setting and manipulating your media tags even easier than title and description tags. You don't even need to install a plugin to perform his next step.

First, click on Pages and Add New in the left hand pane of your WordPress dashboard or click Edit under the title of a page that you have already created. Once in the creation or editing page, you will notice a small button at the top left corner of the screen that reads Add Media. Click on that now.

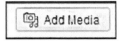

Here you can upload media from a drive of your choice or you can enter the URL of a media file from elsewhere on the web. Once you select your media, you will be taken to a section of the page that asks you to enter specific data about that media file.

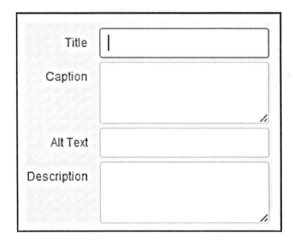

Here is where you will set the media file's name or title, a caption, alt text and a description. The title of your media file should be named after your keywords. So if you just uploaded an image that depicted a dental implant on our Dental Implants page, your title might be dental-implants-austin-tx.jpg.

We recommend that you name your media files just like that, with small letters and separated by spaces for ease of identification and organization. We also recommend organizing your media files and their metadata attributes on a spreadsheet file just like you did with your page titles and descriptions. In other words, record and keep track of everything for easy recall later.

The caption you enter will show up on your web page underneath the visible file in question, and you are encouraged to use keywords in your captions for further on-page SEO. Your description of the above example image might be, "Dental implants: a viable alternative to dentures for our treasured Austin patients."

Alt text is the text that will show up on text-only browsers or that will be read aloud to the hearing impaired. Remember, the search engines can't see your images and videos. They can only judge their relevancy by the metadata that you enter. Your alt text should describe your images and videos and should also include your keywords for best results. Alt Text entered for the above Dental Implant image might read, "A close up image of a dental implant from our Austin, TX office."

The description you enter will be used in search engine image searches. This should be written in the same vein as page descriptions. Your example might read, "At GenericDental in Austin, Texas, we use the highest-quality and most realistic looking dental implants. Make an appointment today!"

Optimize all of your media files this way and you will get a leg up in the SERPs for all relevant searches.

Header-Tags

When writing the text content on your individual pages, we earlier recommended that you break up the content with bolded subheaders and bullet points wherever possible. This makes the page easier on the eyes and the content much easier to digest; but organizing your site in this manner also improves SEO.

When separating your content with bolded subheaders, use relevant Header-tags. These can be selected by using the paragraph drop down box in the page editor.

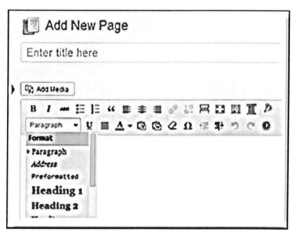

Using Heading 1, Heading 2, Heading 3 and so on for your headings and subheadings will tell the search engines that those terms are crucial and thus they should be taken into account when ranking your site in the SERPs. Knowing this, you are encouraged to use your keywords in your Header or H-Tags whenever possible.

For instance, right above a paragraph about dental implants, we might use the Heading 1 attribute to write the heading, "High-Quality Dental Implants – The Best in Austin," assuming that those terms represent one or more of your primary keywords.

Valuable Content

The search engines are becoming more intelligent every day and they can determine if you have written content just to write or if you have strived to provide your future visitors with the very best content they can find online.

To achieve stellar search engine rankings, you need to be able to inform, educate and entertain. You need to answer your web visitors' questions and you need to provide more or better information than your competitors are offering. This requires extensive research and great writing abilities, or you can hire a professional like we recommended in previous sections.

Low Keyword Density

We mentioned that inserting your keywords into your web content is crucial for achieving high rankings, but we also cautioned against keywords stuffing. Your job is to use just enough keywords to appease the search engines while alleviating them of doubt that you are trying to game the system.

For best results, we recommend using your keyword in your page's title, once in the first paragraph, once in the final paragraph and a couple of times throughout the page (utilizing H-tag keywords whenever possible).

This should provide your page with a keyword density of 1-3%, which is ideal for on-page SEO. To find your keyword density, calculate the word count of the page you have written and then count the number of keywords you used. Then divide the keyword amount by the word count to find your keyword density. So your calculation may look like this: 5 keywords/500 words = .01 or 1% Keyword Density.

Keep in mind that you may be using multiple keywords on a single page. The keyword density should be calculated for each keyword that you use for best results.

Internal Linking Structure

An internal linking structure is crucial in making your website more user-friendly. Visitors to your site don't always want to click on your main menu to find the content they need. When they stumble across particular keywords in your web content, such as Dental Implants, they may appreciate a link to your Implants page. Not only will providing internal links make your site easier to navigate, but it helps the search engines determine which keywords are the most important to rank you for.

To create internal links, edit one of your already-created web pages or posts and find a keyword within the content. Highlight the keyword and click on the Link icon in your page edit toolbar.

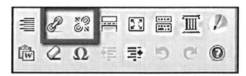

Notice how there are two icons. The first icon sets the link and the second icon removes a link in case you created one erroneously. Once you have highlighted the keyword and clicked on the link icon, you will be taken to a pop-up page that asks for the preferred link URL.

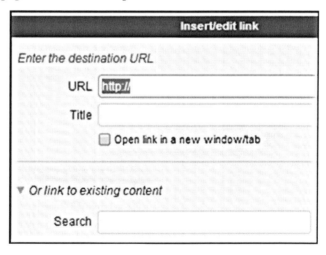

Here you can either enter a new URL if you want to provide an external link or you can search within your own pages to provide an internal link. Since you are creating an internal link, you will want to find the page within your site that is relevant to the keyword you have just selected, such as your Dental Implants page.

The rules of internal linking are to keep it to one or maybe two inter⬚
per page. More than that and your page may appear to be too clutter⬚
should also ensure that the pages you link to are in fact relevan⬚ ⬚⬚ ⬚⬚⬚
keyword in question. Ask yourself if linking to that page will make your site
more user-friendly or if it will only lead to the frustration of your web
visitors. Remember that you are helping your visitors more easily navigate
your page, and you should approach internal linking while keeping that in
mind.

Site Map

Even though the search engines can crawl your site and all of its pages in a
matter of seconds (or even fractions of a second), they will always appreciate
any help you can provide them with. One way you can help the search
engines crawl your website and all of its pages is to provide them with an
easy-to-crawl site map.

A site map is a coded document that showcases every link on your site in
the order of their importance. This way the search engines can go from link
to link and page to page, ensuring that they have found everything there is
to index and rank.

Creating a site map for your website is easy with the help of a site called xml-
sitemaps (www.xml-sitemaps.com).

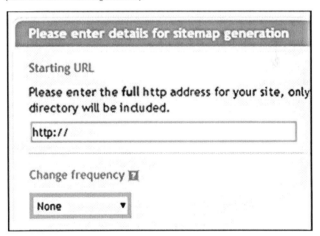

Here you will enter your website's domain name, the frequency with which
you want the search engines to crawl your site, the last modification
attribute, your priority preference and that's it. Click start and you're off to
completing your on-site SEO.

For our purposes, we recommend that you just enter your domain, hit start and keep all the other options in their default positions. Once you have this document, you will be wise to submit your site map to Google Webmaster Tools. This basically tells Google that your site is ready to be indexed.

Keep in mind that, due to the steps we have already taken, Google will crawl your website even if you don't submit it to the search engine for the purposes of indexing. By submitting your site to Google Webmaster Tools, you are taking a proactive step that tells Google that your site is ready for indexing now rather than later.

Visit Webmaster Tools:

https://www.google.com/webmasters/tools/home?hl=en

Then enter your website when prompted. Once your website is set up, click on your website name, then under the heading Crawl, locate the Sitemaps link.

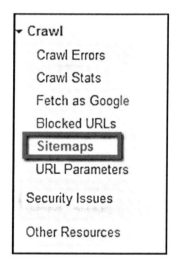

In the upper right hand corner, you will notice a button that says Add/Test Sitemap. Click on that button, add your xml sitemap and you're done. Well, almost.

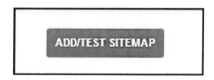

We also recommend that you place your site map in the footer of your website, for ease of use by visitors and search engines alike. Most footer plugins will make it easy to insert your site map and other elements into your footer, such as social buttons and important links, such as your Privacy Policy and Terms and Conditions, which are important for legal reasons.

| Emergency Dental |Testimonials| About |Dentist News| Contact Us| Privacy Policy | Site Map
Copyright © 2014 Mint Dental. All rights reserved -
Website & Marketing by Firegang Digital Marketing

On-Site SEO - Not Just For Web Pages

Knowing what you now do about on-site optimization, you can apply that knowledge to all web content, including your blog and social media accounts. Since your blog is connected to your WordPress website, creating your title and description tags, media tags and H-tags can be applied to every blog entry you publish.

Your social media accounts are handled a bit differently. While most social content isn't indexed by the Google, Google+ content is. Furthermore, each platform, such as Facebook, has its own powerful internal search engine that users may utilize to find your practice. Keep this fact in mind when filling out your profiles and optimize accordingly.

To apply on-site SEO to social media profiles, think of your name as your title tag, your About or Story as your description, your media titles and descriptions as media tags and your content as the valuable content and H-tags.

A Final Word About Quality

We feel that it is important to offer a word of warning about on-site SEO. You can become so focused on optimizing your site and all of its content for ease-of-crawling by automated bots that you can completely forget about your human audience. Don't do this. The rule is, optimize for your prospects and patients first and the search engines second. Use these tips, keep that rule in mind, and your site will not only provide value, but you will likely rank prominently also.

***

Off-Site (Off Page) SEO - Establishing the Authority of Your Web Presence

You could have perfect on-site SEO and you still might not experience the rankings you hope to achieve. That is because Google and the other search engines are wary of sites that have perfect on-site SEO and poor off-site SEO.

Off-site SEO, to the search engines, means that others vouch for your site. It represents social proof, and without it, Google and the other engines may ignore your site altogether, no matter how perfect your on-site SEO happens to be.

The search engines use two primary factors to determine social proof: backlinks and social sharing. Backlinks, as you now know, are external links that point from other websites to yours. For example, the Better Business Bureau linking to your site means that your site must be a pretty good business with a great reputation in your local community. Social sharing indicates that others have shared your website, pages and other content with their social followers and friends.

The more relevant external links you have and the more social sharing your content experiences, the more your rankings should improve, as long as those links and social shares were gained legitimately.

Again, Google and the other engines are wary of sites that gain too many backlinks too quickly or that suddenly accumulate thousands of social network friends and shares seemingly overnight. To avoid sending up a red flag and to keep Google and the other engines rewarding you for your hard work, you are encouraged to gain outside links and social shares organically and naturally. This can be accomplished by using the following tips.

Tips to Improve Off-Site SEO

Contact Partners and Relevant Organizations: If you belong to the American Dental Association, the Better Business Bureau, the local Chamber of Commerce or others, contact those entities and ask for your website to be linked-to from their websites and social media profiles.

Social Sharing: Place social buttons next to your blog posts and on your website to make it easy for visitors to share your content on Facebook, Twitter, Google+ and any other social accounts they may use. Many WordPress plugins can accomplish this. You can improve off-site SEO by sharing your pages and posts on your own social accounts where you can then encourage others to pass your content around.

Review Sites: Platforms like Yelp, Angie's List and FourSquare invite others to relay their personal experiences with businesses just like yours.

Invite your patients to visit these sites and leave their own reviews for improved off-site SEO. We will explain this in further detail in a coming section.

The Key is to Look for Sustainable Results

While other webmasters are trying to game Google's system in the hopes of receiving instant and massive results, you are encouraged to use this advice to look for gradual but longer lasting results. Put the preceding steps into place and you will experience just that.

Chapter 9: Local Search Engine Optimization

Many of the SEO tricks that we have taught you thus far are designed for global search optimization. This essentially means that your website, blog and social media accounts will be able to be located by people searching for your keyword terms no matter where they happen to be located in the world. But your practice isn't really interested in being found globally. You rely on local customers to keep your business solvent and growing every year, so this section will show you how to optimize strictly for a local audience.

The search engines, and Google in particular, have been putting much focus into local search for quite a few years now. If you are searching from a desktop or laptop computer, Google will detect what location you are searching from and will do its best to yield local results whenever possible. And now with GPS devices in most phones and mobile devices, providing search customers with local results is even easier. As a local SEO professional, your job is to tell Google and the other search engines exactly where to rank you so that your practice shows up for relevant and localized prospects and patients. This is where Local SEO comes into play.

How Local SEO is Different

To see how a global search result looks, try searching Google for the keyword term, "Dental staff training tips".

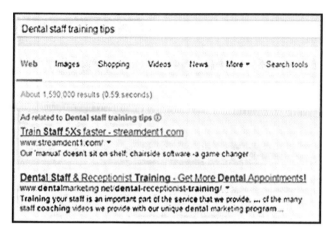

Notice how Google delivers results from all over the web. You might even notice a video or two that could have been filmed and uploaded from anywhere.

Now look at what happens when you enter a geographical modifier into the mix. This time, conduct a search for "Dentures in Austin, Texas".

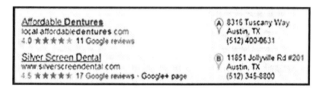

Notice how Google not only yields results from Austin, Texas, but you are even provided with a map so that you can gauge which dentures provider is closest to where you are located.

By now you already know how to enter your geographic modifiers into your keywords, and thus you already have some knowledge of local SEO. We are going to expand on that knowledge so that you can completely dominate your local area within the search engines, including Google and any others your prospects and patients happen to be using.

Entering your physical location – city, state, burb names, etc. – is only half the battle when it comes to local SEO. The true determination of how well you rank in local SEO depends on your use of your practice's Citations.

Citations & Their Importance in Local SEO Rankings

A citation is a snippet of data that the search engines use to learn more about your practice, location, services, hours of operation and other important details. At its core, your practice's citations consist of your NAP, which as you know by now is your office Name, Address and Phone Number.

Take a look at your search results for the Austin, Texas dentist. Notice how you have names, addresses and phone numbers on each. Those are citations at work.

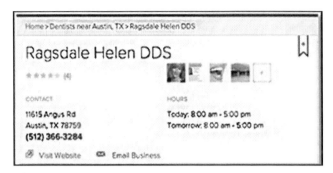

It is crucial that your citations be correct and consistent across the web. Just as the search engines crawl your site for information, they are also crawling millions of other sites across the web from all over the world. Ideally, you will want your practice's citations to be listed on your own website and on other prominent websites, such as the Better Business Bureau, Dunn and Bradstreet and the local Chamber of Commerce. The more citations you have listed online – as long as those citations are correct and consistent – the more clout your online presence will be said to have and the higher you will theoretically rank in the local search results.

Mapping Services

In a moment, we are going to teach you how to build your citations across the web so that your practice can enjoy the social clout and high rankings we have just discussed. Having your citations prominently displayed in hundreds or thousands of places online not only makes your practice seem important, but it will also make your practice very easy to find for prospects and patients who may be using mapping and GPS services to find your office location.

Before you start to build your citations across the web, you need to make sure that any platforms that currently list your practice are showcasing the most accurate information. The platforms to check include such pages as Insider Pages, Yellowpages.com, City Search and many, many others. Instead of visiting each page one-by-one for the purposes of verifying your information, we are going to teach you a little shortcut.

Step 1: Check Your Citation Information Across the Web

If your practice has any information listed on one or more online directories, and chances are you do if you have been at your location for some time, you are likely to find inconsistencies. For example, Yahoo may display a phone number and address that is no long valid, such as if you recently moved locations. You may find bad office hours on Yelp; and if you recently purchased a new domain name and created a new website like we instructed you to in the beginning of this book, you will need to alter your URL on every single directory that lists your practice's information online.

To find out whether the information listed on the web is correct or not, we are going to recommend two important platforms: Yext and Whitespark.

Yext (www.yext.com)

Yext is a service that will allow you to search for your practice's citations across the web absolutely free. Simply add your name, business name and phone number and click Scan Now to get started.

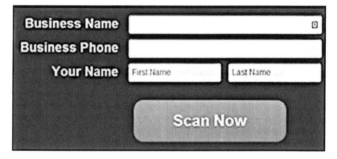

When the scan has finished, you will see a list of online directories, social media sites, online forums and other platforms that may potentially list your practice information. You will also be able to see exactly which errors need to be fixed. At the top of the page, you will be provided with a number, which represents the number of errors that Yext has found.

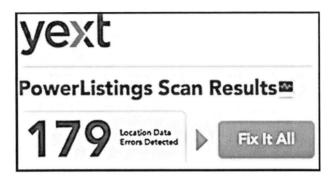

We recommend that you use this free report and begin to fix your citations one-by-one across the web. Yext will do the work for you, for a fee of course, but if you are looking to keep costs down, you would be better served correcting this information manually.

WhiteSpark (whitespark.ca/local-citation-finder)

Whitespark is like Yext on steroids. The company offers a host of SEO tools, but we are primarily interested in the local citation finder.

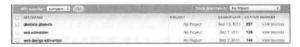

This tool will search for your citations across the web, notify you of errors and so much more. In fact, Whitespark will allow you to analyze and monitor your citations to improve accuracy over time, something that Yext doesn't do.

For best results, we recommend using both tools in order to receive a thorough report informing you of where your Citations dispersal campaign needs work.

***

Step 2: Correct Your Citation Information with the Big 3 Data Aggregators

If you have just run a Yext and/or Whitespark citation report and you have found your citations on a few local online directories, social networks and other sites, you may wonder how the information got there if you didn't submit yourself. Online directories like MapQuest, Yellow Pages and even Google+ Business 'scrape' your practice information from authority sources; and those sources are where you should start if you want to control, correct and maintain the most accurate information online.

If online directories had a hierarchy, at the top of the hierarchy would be the big three data aggregators. If you have information listed online and you didn't enter it yourself, chances are that it came from one of these three sites. Let's examine these sites now so that you can edit any information that needs to be corrected before you proceed.

InfoGroup

(http://expressupdateusa.com)

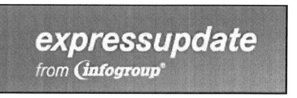

To populate or correct your practice information within InfoGroup for the purposes of spreading it far and wide online, start with the section reserved for Small Business Owners. Simply click on Go to New Site and you will be presented with a search box at the top of the page. Enter your business name and your citation search will begin.

If your practice's name is unique, your business should show up as the first and only listing in the search results. Click on Claim Now. If your practice name is shared by others across the country, you may see a list of practices to choose from. Select your practice and click Claim Now.

You will be asked to verify your listing via phone. The site will first ask you if your listed phone number is correct and, if it is, you will receive a phone call to verify.

If you don't see your practice listed, scroll to the bottom of the page and click on the link Add it Now.

Add or edit your site as instructed and you will receive an email from www.expressupdateusa.com when the listing is considered in review.

Acxiom

(www.databyacxiom.com)

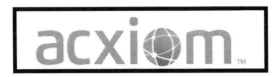

When landing on the Acxiom Home page, just like you did with InfoGroup, click on the link for small business owners titled Get Started to do just that.

On the next page, you will see several options. We recommend that you click the link that is specified for small business owners with one or a few locations.

Next, you will be asked to search for your business by phone number in order to claim and correct any information listed. Do that now.

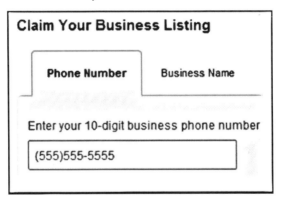

You will then be able to edit your practice information or add your business for the purposes of mass aggregation.

Localeze (www.neustarlocaleze.biz/directory/search)

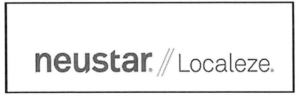

When you land on the Localeze site, you will be asked to search for your practice by your business name and zip code or your city and state. You also have the option of searching by phone number.

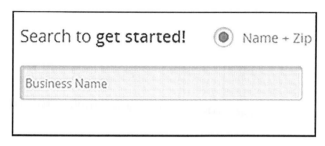

Whether you add or edit your information, you will be asked to verify your listing by phone, just like you did with the other two aggregator sites.

Once you have finished adding or correcting your information on the big three aggregators, your information will soon make it to many more online directories, social media sites, forums and more platforms across the web. But you don't want to quit now. To be extra thorough, you will want to move on to the next tier of aggregators to further improve your local SEO clout.

***

Step 3: Inspect Other Key Online Directories

Your Yext and/or Whitespark reports will likely show the following sites. We recommend that you start with these before you proceed to any others if you want an accurate and consistent web presence.

Google+ Business

(http://www.google.com/+/business/)

Considered the king of local SEO platforms and a must for local SEO domination, Google+ Business will help you gain prominent local rankings. Your practice will also show up for all relevant searches on Google Maps. Since you already have a profile on this platform, you already have a leg up when it comes to local search engine optimization.

Bing Places for Business

(https://www.bingplaces.com)

While Google is considered the number one search engine in the world, Bing is quickly catching up as number two. Microsoft's search engine also provides a local place for small business owners, and you are encouraged to fill out your Bing Places with all of the information you used to populate your Google+ Business account for best results.

Yahoo Small Business

(http://smallbusiness.yahoo.com/local-listings/basic-listing)

Yahoo, the third largest search engine in the world, also provides a local place. If you visit Yahoo Small business and you find your practice but the information is incorrect, we recommend that you create a fresh listing, wait for that one to go live and then request that the incorrect listing be removed.

Yelp

(http://www.yelp.com)

Yelp is where people go when they want to leave a review on a particular business, such as your dental practice. Creating a profile on Yelp invites others to leave their reviews about your services, and that is a very good thing. As you will read in the next section, and as we've mentioned previously, most people today view online reviews as being equal to a personal recommendation from a friend, relative or neighbor.

City Search

(http://www.citysearch.com/world)

Adding and editing listings on City Search, which used to be the go-to place for finding anything local, and still is for many individuals, has always been a little tricky. We recommend that you contact the administrators via email if you run into any problems. The platform is usually good about responding to queries and fixing whatever needs to be fixed.

Yellow Pages

(http://www.yellowpages.com)

Remember those big yellow books that decimated entire forests that people used to find local businesses, addresses and phone numbers? Today, people in search of contact information simply have to visit YellowPages.com. Make sure your business is listed and correct so that customers can find you and so that any other aggregators receiving information from this ultra-respected online source have the true and correct information.

Super Pages

(http://www.superpages.com)

Similar to Yellow Pages, Super Pages is another online directory that is still used by many humans and aggregators alike.

Angie's List

(http://www.angieslist.com)

Kind of like a cross between Craig's List and Yelp, Angie's List is a platform where local customers can go to find profiles, advertisements and online reviews for many local businesses. Many people use Angie's List to find dental professionals, so don't leave Angie off of your list of databases and review sites to use.

Mojo Pages

(http://www.mojopages.com)

This site advertises that customers can find local businesses in half the time, but that won't be the case at all if your practice name isn't listed and you fail to control your online information. You will also be happy to know that many local TV stations use Mojo Pages to provide data for their Yellow Pages sections.

Local.com

(http://www.local.com)

If you look at the bottom of Local, which is a very prestigious local data aggregator, you will notice that it reads, "Some data provided by Acxiom," which you now know is one of the big three data aggregators online. Your data may already be correct on Local since you added or edited your site on Acxiom, but check your information on the platform just to be sure.

Kudzu

(http://www.kudzu.com)

Kudzu mentions that it gets most of its information from Localeze. Again, check to see if your practice is listed on Kudzu just in case.

Yellow Bot

(http://www.yellowbot.com)

Another Yellow Pages directory to list your citations. Hey, as far as data aggregators go, the more the merrier.

Yellow Book

(www.yellowbook.com)

When you add your information to Yellow Book, prospects and patients will be able to find your phone number, address and a map to your location. They can also click a link that allows them to receive a call from your practice.

Four Square

(https://foursquare.com)

This platform allows users to check-in to your practice using their smartphones and leave reviews. We will be using this platform in the next section, so make sure your profile is filled out.

Merchant Circle

(http://www.merchantcircle.com)

Another site that used to be the go-to for local products and services, Merchant Circle can give you another local space to advertise your dental practice.

MapQuest

(http://www.mapquest.com)

MapQuest used to be the go-to map service before Google and Apple came along. Despite it dropping in popularity, the platform still holds its authority in many respects.

***

Add, edit and claim your information on all of the above directories and you will provide Google and the other search engines with the information they need to rank you prominently and drive prospects and patients your way.

Now it is time to discuss reputation management and online reviews, the next section of your dental Internet marketing campaign.

Chapter 10: Reputation Management & Online Reviews

Your practice is already familiar with offline reputation management. This is that word-of-mouth advertising and over-the-water-cooler scuttlebutt that can make or break your business, depending on what word-on-the-street has to say about your practice.

You can do some things to control your offline reputation, such as providing excellent products and services, treating your patients with respect and by making sure the office and dental environment is clean and organized.

Online reputation management works a bit differently. While much of offline reputation management is out of your control, you can actually control and manage your online reputation so that your practice is always presented in the best light. This is what we are going to show you how to do right now.

Online reputation management largely centers around online reviews. Those are the reviews we mentioned on sites like Google+ Business, Yelp, Angie's List and Four Square that help prospects and patients choose your practice over the competition. It's said that 89% of users trust online reviews and that number is only expected to rise as more people take to the Internet to find the products and services they desire most.

By populating the Internet with positive reviews about your practice from actual patients that you have done business with, you can succeed in bringing more prospects and patients into your office. Not only that, but more positive reviews can also help with local search engine optimization.

While positive reviews can help your business, it is only logical to assume that negative reviews will harm it. Consider this statistic. It is said that for every negative review your practice earns, you can potentially lose 30 patients. That figure might mean that thirty patients skip over your practice when deciding on a dental professional, or it could indicate thirty patients leaving your practice for another dentist in the area. Either way, we are going to help you avoid negative reviews whenever possible. And if you do happen to receive a negative review, we are going to teach you how to negate that review so that the harm it does is minimal or nonexistent.

Where to Gather Online Reviews

Your job, if you want more positive reviews for your practice, is to make it very easy for current patients to leave their experiences and deepest inner thoughts. We recommend that you do this directly from your website first and foremost.

Step 1: Create a Review Us Page for your Website

The first step to encouraging online reviews is to create a new page on your WordPress website. The page you create will consist of nothing more than icons from today's top review sites along with buttons that contain strong calls-to-action like, "Leave a Review!"

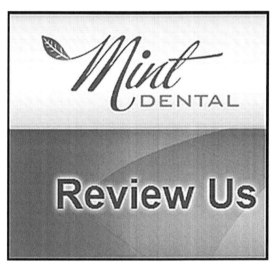

Once that page is completed, tell all of your current patients about it. This can occur before their appointments as they are checking in, during their appointments or as they are settling their accounts prior to leaving your office.

The more people you ask, the more reviews you are likely to receive. While you should never ask for a positive review, it never hurts to tell your patients to relay to others how much they love the practice, or something to that effect. Of course, the reality of the situation is, patients of yours are going to leave the reviews they want to leave. Hopefully most or all of them are positive in nature.

The first of your profiles to link to is Google+ Business, which has the greatest potential to contribute to more prominent local search results. . When you receive online reviews on Google+ Business, your rating level will actually show up in your local search results.

To see this phenomenon in action, conduct a local search for a dentist, such as using the keywords, "Dentist in Houston".

Midtown Dentistry
midtowndentistry.com
4.9 ★★★★★ 113 Google reviews · Google+ page

Charles Sutherland, DDS
www.downtowndentist.com
4.2 ★★★★☆ 5 Google reviews · Google+ page

The University of Texas School of Dentistry...
dentistry.uth.edu
3.9 ★★★★☆ 6 Google reviews · Google+ page

Urban Dental
www.urban-dental.com
2 Google reviews · Google+ page

Royal Dental
www.royaldentalusa.com
4.2 ★★★★☆ 31 Google reviews · Google+ page

Notice how some dentists have yellow stars in their listings and some dental professionals possess more stars than others? It turns out, those dentists with more stars next to their names may also be earning more patients. That star rating system is connected to the practice's Google+ Business account. The more positive reviews you gather on Google+ Business, the more stars your practice will receive on its local search listings.

For a more attractive search presence that you hope your prospects and patients will respond to, send your customers to Google+ Business first and then to Yahoo Places, Insider Pages, Yelp, Four Square and any others you wish to optimize.

Of course, for best results, you can ask patients to leave reviews on every site you create a Review Us button for. Whether that will happen remains up to them, but it never hurts to ask.

***

Step 2: Use Positive Reviews to Their Maximum Advantage

The moment a positive review comes in, you will want to respond to it. Thank patients for leaving their thoughts and tell them that you can't wait to see them back in your office. Responding to reviews shows your audience that you are paying attention, listening and it may encourage others to leave their thoughts when they otherwise may have passed on the opportunity.

Be sure to thank the patient online and in the office for their excellent contribution and be sure to thank and reward them on your social media accounts to show others just how well you treat your very best patients.

If you are worried about responding to online reviews out of fear of revealing personal information or violating HIPAA and any local/state privacy laws, here are the three rules for responding to reviews that you are encouraged to teach to your staff and follow.

1. Never discus patient names or personal details publically unless you have received written permission from your patients to do so.
2. Be general when giving advice and about your general commitment to the overall well-being and care of your patients' oral health.
3. Think long and hard about how to respond before you commit. Once your response is live, there is no going back.
4. Take the situation offline by telling the patient that you would love to discuss the matter in private and then leave your phone number for the person to call.

***

Step 3: Mitigate Any Damage Negative Reviews May Cause

In a perfect world, your practice would receive nothing but the very best reviews people can leave. Unfortunately, this isn't a perfect world and your practice is likely to receive at least one bad review that causes your stomach to knot up and that sets your mind racing, wondering if this one negative comment could ruin your practice altogether. Here are nine steps to follow if and when that time comes.

1. **Respond in a Timely Manner:** The moment a negative review comes in, forget about the potential thirty patients you might lose and take time to respond to the person who left the review in question.

2. **Be Brief:** If you respond with more than two sentences, you can come across as being defensive. It is best to keep it quick and to the point.

3. **Be Empathetic:** Let the reviewer know that you know exactly what he or she is going through and that you want nothing more than to ensure their satisfaction. Get a dialogue started and find out what is truly bothering the person in question. For good measure, make sure you thank the person for leaving the review he or she left.

4. **Offer Something of Value:** Gauge what you feel the reviewer most wants and provide it, either in the form of a free offer, discount or complete refund. The small amount of money you lose on the act of turning a negative comment into a positive one could earn your practice thousands more later on.

5. **Know When to Say When:** Do not get into a heated debate with a patient online, especially if the person leaving the negative review resorts to ad hominem attacks or starts making impossible demands, such as urging you to fire of one of your staff members. To handle situations like these, tell the reviewer that you are sorry for their dissatisfaction; that you will do whatever it takes to make it right, and then ask to speak to the person in private. Leave your phone number and then leave it alone.

6. **Ask to Get Them Removed:** There is always a chance that the platform in question – Google, for example – will remove negative reviews, if there is good reason for it, such as if the comment is from an online troll.

7. **Don't Feed the Trolls:** Keep in mind that there are essentially two types of negative reviews. There are truthful ones where a patient is relaying an experience that actually happened and then there are troll reviews. Troll reviews may or may not be truthful and they may not even come from current patients, but the reviews themselves are almost always designed to hurt your practice in some way.

An example might be, "Doctor Peters ripped my teeth out without anesthetic and then charged me $5,000 for it."

Even if the negative comment is ridiculous and fills you with rage, respond professionally and with good humor and let the person know that you will fix the problem however possible. The object of a troll is to get you to respond with vitriol. This will not only show your practice in a bad light, but you might lose even more patients with your anger and off-kilter language than the negative review could ever hope to.

While you can try to get troll reviews removed, most of them will remain. It is best to just roll with the punches and have faith that more positive reviews are just around the corner.

8. **Use Negativity to Improve:** It is best to discuss negative reviews with your staff during regular meetings. Decide what comments are truthful and what can be improved upon and use that information to make your practice and the staff who run it even better.

9. **Bury Negative Reviews:** The only way you can truly minimize or omit the damage done from negative reviews is to ensure that no one sees them. Call your current patients – your very best ones – and ask them to leave a review. The more positive reviews you receive, the more of your negative ones you will bury. Just make sure that you optimize your practice, treatments and patient services so that you get far more positive reviews than negative, if you happen to get any negative reviews at all.

***

Now it is time to discuss the very best way to dominate the local SERPs that doesn't involve organic search engine optimization. We are talking about, of course, paid search advertising. With the proper budget and the following advice, your ads will show up for relevant users anytime they search for your keywords. Your job is to entice them to click-through your ads, to call, email or come in for a face-to-face visit. We will now show you how to do just that.

Chapter 11: Pay-Per-Click Search Engine Advertising

You will now learn how to use paid search ads, which accompany the organic listings on the right hand and upper portions of the SERPs, to their maximum advantage. The type of advertising that we are going to focus on is known as PPC marketing or pay-per-click. This is the type of advertising that Google uses to monetize its search engine. By monetizing search with the PPC model, Google has effectively become one of the wealthiest and most successful companies in the history of the world. This is how the advertising model works.

Google Adwords

Before you get started with Adwords, it is important for you to understand that spending money on PPC does not guarantee results; and doing so doesn't even guarantee that your ads will show up for relevant searches. When a search user enters one of your keywords into their Google search box, Adwords will determine which advertisers have set the highest bids for the keyword in question.

If your bid outshines all the others who may be optimizing for the same keyword, your ads will show up first and that increases the potential that they will be clicked. Your job is to create ads that are extra-enticing, so that prospects and patients are quick-to-click.

You will then be charged a certain amount each time your ads are clicked. The amount you are charged per click depends on the competitiveness of the keyword in question. The more competitive the keyword, the higher the charge to your Adwords account.

This is why it is essential that you set a daily budget, so that you don't exhaust your total budget the very first day your ads are run. Once your daily budget has been reached, your ads will disappear from rotation for that day until the very next day when your ads and daily budget will start all over again.

That is the Adwords PPC advertising model in a nutshell. In this section, we are going to show you step-by-step how to set up an Adwords account and prepare your first campaign to go live. Don't worry, all basic settings and preference choices will be explained, and we will also briefly touch on the more advanced options just in case you want to take your PPC performance to the next level.

A Word About Results

Many dental professionals come to us after already attempting a PPC campaign where they experienced little to no results. This leaves them with a bad taste in their mouths that the strongest mint toothpaste couldn't hope to put a dent in.

If you have had a previously bad experience with PPC marketing, we ask that you give it one more shot using the steps we have outlined below. While immediate results certainly are possible, we ask that you give it at least three months to show the results you are hoping for. Later in this section, we will teach you how to analyze and test various data points to further optimize your PPC campaign and enhance the results you experience.

Step 1: Set Up a Google Adwords Account

First visit the Google Adwords home page (https://adwords.google.com) and sign in using your Google+ account information that you were provided with earlier. Once you are in, Google will ask you a series of questions, such as your country, time zone and the currency that you would like to use for your PPC campaign.

Once you have completed that step and you have confirmed your account, you will be prepared to create your first Campaign and Ad Group.

Proper Organization is the Key to Adwords Success

Your PPC account should be structured in order from broader campaign ideas to more narrowed-down ad groups and keywords. This is known as campaign segmenting. Just as you were advised to segment your email list into groups of prospects, patients and former patients, for example, we advise that you organize your PPC campaigns the same exact way.

You might segment your campaigns based on the products and treatments that you offer or the general location of your practice. You may segment your campaigns based on how well they perform, or how poorly, or how much you have set to bid for certain keywords. This segment hierarchy is completely up to you, but it is recommended that you organize your account properly for better results. Proper organization will also allow for easier testing later on. We recommend creating another tab in your spreadsheet to keep track of all Adwords campaigns, ad groups and keywords.

A sample ad campaign may seek to build awareness and drive conversions for dental implants. The campaign titled Dental Implants might then have ad groups that focus on partial implants, full implants, implant dentures, and so on. You might then have another ad group titled Teeth Whitening with ad groups that focus on in-office teeth whitening, take-home teeth whitening kits and laser teeth whitening.

The ad groups you set can then have an infinite number of ads; it all depends on the keywords you hope to optimize for and the budgets you have in place.

We recommend that you set 3-5 ad groups per campaign for easy maintenance. You can always create more, but we find this number to be the sweet spot, especially when you have many ad groups running simultaneously. And if your practice offers ten or more services, with 3-5 ad groups running per service, you will have plenty on your plate to deal with. Don't become overwhelmed. We will show you how to easily maintain, optimize and supercharge your PPC campaigns once they go live.

***

Step 2: Create Your First Campaign

To create your very first campaign, click on the Campaigns tab near the top of the page and find the Add Campaign button.

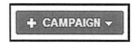

When you click on that button, you will be asked to specify the network you wish for your ads to be displayed on. We recommend that you select the option Search Network with Display Select.

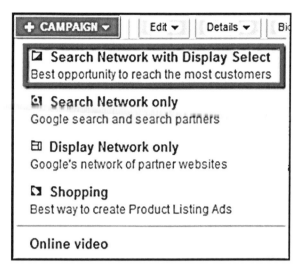

As Google suggests, this is the best opportunity to reach the most customers. The other options do have their merits, but for beginners and until you can learn the intricacies of the Adwords mechanism, it is best to keep things broad in order to maximize the effectiveness of the ads that you are about to create.

Ad Campaign Settings

Here you will be asked to name your first campaign. We recommend that you select a product or service, such as Tooth Extractions. Keep the type of ad and the Network settings in their default positions for now. Again, you can always change these at a later date.

Devices: We recommend that you keep the default setting for devices, which indicates that all of your ads will properly show up for all types of devices, from computers to tablets. Later on you will learn how to test your results to find out how your prospects and patients are finding and landing on your online presence. If you find that most of your visitors are using tablet computers to access your site, for example, you will want to come back to this setting in the future and select 'Tablets with full browsers' when prompted.

Locations: Here is where you should set your local area, since you rely on local customers first and foremost. Select the radio button 'Let me Choose' and enter all the geographic modifiers that your audience might use to find your practice.

156

On the other hand, if you are selling products through your website to a national and even worldwide audience, this is where you will alter the settings to reflect those changes. Then select the languages that you would like your ads to be optimized for.

Bid Strategy: This is where you will tell Adwords how you wish to bid for the keywords you want to optimize for. We recommend that you keep the default setting 'I'll manually set my bids for clicks'. This is where you will set a maximum cost-per-click or CPC for each keyword in question. Your daily budget will then never be charged over that amount for any single click.

The other option is to have Adwords set your bids, which could turn out to be an outrageous amount, depending on the competitive nature of the keyword in question. For right now, set your own bids and reserve allowing Adwords to do it once you have gained more experience with the PPC advertising model.

Default Bid: This is the maximum bid amount you will be willing to pay for the first ad group in your campaign. We recommend that you set this low for now, say $3, until you have more data to justify bidding higher amounts. You can always change this amount later.

Daily Budget: This is the maximum amount you are willing to spend on your pay-per-click ads on any given day. For example, if your bid amount is $5 and your daily limit is $10, your ads can be clicked two times before your ads disappear from the network until the next day, whereby your daily budget will start over again.

The minimum amount Google allows is $10. We recommend that you divide your total budget by the amount of days in the month so that you can maximize your click allowance and, as you will soon learn how to do, improve your ad conversions.

Ad Extensions: We recommend that you select all three ad extensions offered to you by Adwords. Doing so will allow you to show your location, web addresses to specific pages on your site and your phone number directly in your ads. In theory, prospects who then see your ads won't even have to click-through to your website in order to convert.

***

Step 3: Create Your First Ad Group

Set your Ad Group name, which should be a subset of your campaign category, such as Veneers under the campaign Cosmetic Dentistry.

Now you will create your ad. To help you create the most engaging ads possible, put these Adwords ad creation best practices to good use.

Character Limits: You are only allowed 25 characters for the headline, 35 characters for description lines one and two, 35 characters for the display URL and 1042 characters for the actual URL that you want to set.

With so little space allowed, it is wise to learn to be very good at condensing your ideas into just a few words or less.

Stand Apart: Take a look at a few of the ads that your competitors have in active rotation. Simply search for your keywords and examine the ads that show up, their titles and ad bodies. You can then click-through to view the landing pages associated with those ads. This research can then be used to make your Adwords ads even more effective.

Promotions, Prices & Special Offers: Your ads will receive a higher amount of conversions, otherwise known as click-throughs, if you mention specific promotions, like Free Teeth Cleanings; prices, like $25 off Teeth Whitening; and special offers, like Refer a Friend and Get $25.

Benefits of Clicking-Through: As concisely as possible and using the small space allotted, you must successfully explain to your audience precisely what they will get out of clicking-through to the landing page you have set out for them to visit.

At Least One Keyword: Include a relevant keyword in your ad at least once, in the title or the body; or both for best results. Don't just include your keywords to include them. They must merge naturally with the other words you have chosen.

Matching Landing Page: Don't just send leads to your home page. You will get far more conversions if you set a dedicated page that is relevant to the ad your prospects are expected to click. This could be your Teeth Whitening webpage for ads in your Teeth Whitening ad group, or you could set a separate dedicated Teeth Whitening page that you will send ad converts to. A dedicated page will be easier to test, since the traffic will come solely from ad click-throughs and thus can be easily experimented with and tweaked to improve results.

Clear Calls-to-Action: As you've learned throughout this book, tell your prospects to call, click, email, submit, buy or come in today! Don't leave their actions up to chance. Tell them what to do directly in your ads and, if you have done everything else correctly, they will gladly comply.

Heed the Rules: You can capitalize the first letters of each word, and you are encouraged to do so to increase conversions, but you should never capitalize every letter of any single word. Don't use excessive punctuation or repeat words for added emphasis, such as Free Free Free; and refrain from using numbers to represent words, such as Braces 4 Less.

Google will penalize you for breaking the rules and this will affect your Adwords Quality Score. The higher your score, the lower you will pay for your ads overall. The lower your score, the more you will pay and the fewer conversions you will experience; making your PPC campaigns ineffective or, worse, useless.

Spend time learning any recently updated rules so that you can avoid penalties or the feared Google Ban Hammer, which will remove your account from the Adwords platform permanently.

URLs: The Display URL is where you will put a shortened domain name, such as your primary domain:

www.GenericDental.com.

The destination URL is the actual domain of the landing page that you will send ad converts to. This can be longer, such as:

www.GenericDental.com/implants/implant-special-offers/coupon-code/.

Ad Extensions: This is where you can offer a downloadable form, phone number, address or special link, as well as a few other capabilities. Choose the ones that you feel will benefit you the most. We recommend that you at least select the phone number, address and email address extensions to increase the number of leads that contact you or come into your office.

***

Step 4: Choose Your Ad Keywords

Here is where you will enter all of the keywords that you want your ads to show up for. You can enter one keyword per line. Choose relevant service keywords, geography keywords and brand keywords, as well as any synonyms and related terms like you learned to do in the keyword research section.

Google also provides a list of suggested keywords based on the name of your campaign and ad group. There is no limit to the amount of keywords you can select, but the more you use the higher the chances that your ads will show up for relevant searches. We recommend including all of the relevant keywords on your list, as well as the ones Google suggests for best results.

***

Step 5: Select Negative Keywords

Adwords allows you to block searches that have nothing to do with your campaigns, ad groups, or keywords. The terms that you wish to block are known as negative keywords. An example might be someone who searches for Dental Clinic in Anchorage. You don't want your ads showing up for people looking for medical clinics, plastic surgery clinics, walk-in clinics, and so on.

You may not know which negative keywords to set right now. Later, you will learn how to analyze your Adwords and overall traffic data. You will also be able to determine what keyword terms search engine users are entering into their search boxes before they click on your ads. If you notice any terms that don't apply, enter them as negative keywords to prevent your ads from showing up for those terms in the future.

***

Step 6: Complete the Adwords Billing Process

You will be asked to set up a credit card, debit card or checking account to fund your Google Adwords account. You can pre-pay your account or you can opt to have Google remove the money from your account at various intervals. Generally speaking, Google will remove payment from your account monthly, unless you set up pre-paid service.

We recommend that you also keep a look out for free Adwords coupons, which offer $100 - or more or less - off of your first Adwords campaign. You will typically receive a coupon in the mail the moment you sign up, but we can't promise anything.

***

Step 7: Expand Your Adwords Campaign

Once you have created your first ad group, continue to create ad groups and set keywords for all of your other products and services that you wish to optimize for. Once those are set, and your billing system is established, your ads will go live. You can check the status of your ads anytime by clicking the Home tab at the top of the Adwords platform.

Home

Here you can view each of your campaigns, ad groups and keywords, as well as how well or poorly they are performing. Right at the top of the page is a breakdown of the data for easy reference.

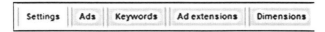

The horizontal bar near the top of the page shows the amount of overall clicks your ads have generated, the impressions they have received – an impression is the amount of times your ads have shown up on individual screens – the click-through rate percentage, the average cost-per-click amount and the overall cost to your Adwords budget.

If you want to manage your campaigns, click on the menu tab of the same name to the right of the Home tab.

Campaigns

Here you will be able to create new campaigns or edit your current ones. You also get a quick snapshot of how each campaign is performing.

Opportunities

Adwords offers you suggestions on how to improve your Adwords campaigns based on the current data. When you first create your campaigns, ad groups and keywords, the Opportunities page will merely explain the service and show a preview for things to come. You will need to wait a while after your PPC campaigns go live to receive the platform's useful and practical advice. We recommend that you check back to the Opportunities tab often to keep up with the latest suggestions Adwords offers.

Tools

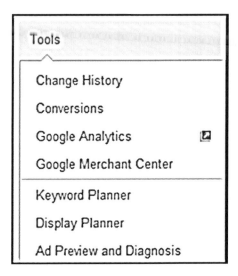

Change History: Here you can view the changes you have applied to your account, as well as edit your account history however you see fit.

Conversions: This tab under Tools allows you to track the keywords that are receiving the most attention – click-throughs, downloads, calls, visits or email forms.

Google Analytics: Google's proprietary web data tracking platform seamlessly merges with Adwords to provide you with even more traffic and conversion data. We will cover Analytics in greater detail in a moment.

Google Merchant Center: This section is for product ads, which you would use if you selected Product Sales when first creating your campaign.

Keyword Planner: We will cover this Adwords Tool in the very next section. You will use it to further hone your keyword list, and further improve your organic and paid search engine optimization efforts.

Display Planner: For image or video ads, Display Ads under Tools will allow you to establish your settings.

Ad Preview and Diagnosis: Click on this tab to search for your ads just as you would in Google. The difference is that you won't be charged for ad impressions as you would if you searched normally. This allows you to check and alter your ads before or during their current rotation.

***

Step 8: Complete Advanced Keyword Research with Google's Keyword Planner

We reserved this section of the book to discuss Google's new keyword research tool. This was due to the fact that Google's Planner, which is the cornerstone of most SEO professionals' keyword strategies, has now merged with the Adwords platform. We felt it appropriate to introduce the tool only after you were familiar with how Adwords operated. Now that you do and now that you have been introduced to the tool, it's time to start utilizing it so that you can hone your current keyword list even further, which – if used properly - will deliver leads like you wouldn't believe.

Imagine finding a keyword that was so highly-searched for, but with such low competition volume that you ranked for it right away. First spot, loud and proud, and receiving tons of visitors and leads to show for it. A situation like that is only possible with the proper and extensive keyword research. So far you know how to brainstorm keywords and you have been provided with a few free and low-cost tools to help you narrow down your list, but Google's Keyword Planner will help to take your organic SEO, local SEO, social marketing and paid marketing efforts to new heights.

Google has created a few keyword research tools in the past. Case in point, the Keyword Tool and Traffic Estimator, two platforms that have been coveted and used for years by webmasters and Internet marketers from all over the world to build and enhance their SEO campaigns. This book will show you how to make the best use of Google's newest creation: The Keyword Planner

Keep in mind that this information could change as time goes on, as technologies become more advanced and as Google alters its business approach. Instead of focusing so much on how to use the platform – which we will of course provide instructions for – pay attention to the ideas behind the how-to's, so that you can roll with the punches and keep the research coming no matter what tools or how much Google alters the Keyword Planner that you will soon become familiar with.

To access the keyword planner, visit your Google Adwords account and click on Tools and then Keyword Planner in the dropdown menu.

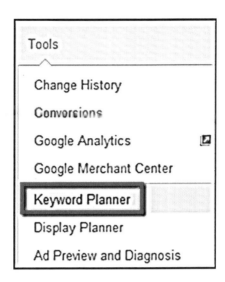

Google Keyword Planner – What it Delivers

Keyword Research: Find out which of your keywords are viable for all of your campaigns by viewing traffic data, competitor data, traffic estimators and more.

Ad Groups: Find out which ad groups are best served to prospects and patients when trying to sell your products and services.

Bids & Budgets: Find out how to set your daily bids and establish budgets based on local trends and competitor data. Keep in mind that these will only be estimates, but they should serve as a guide to propel your Adwords campaign forward.

Match Type: There are three essential type of keyword searches. Broad match, which is characterized by the search term by itself; Exact Match, which is what you are looking for when you put the keyword in brackets; and Phrase Match, which is characterized by quotes on either side of the keyword.

Broad match is like searching for Dentist in Austin and getting results for both Dentist and Austin. This type gives you the most general search results. The search may also include synonyms and related words as Google attempts to understand what you are looking for and yield the best and most accurate results.

You can also use broad match modifiers by using a plus sign in front of words (with no spaces in between like +cosmetic or +implants) to enhance your search, and the results will yield all the sites that use those terms in any order.

Exact Match is like Searching for "Cosmetic Dentist in Atlanta, GA" and getting results for only those sites that were crawled and found to be using that exact term in that exact order and with no other words being used.

Phrase Match is like searching for "Cosmetic dentist in Austin that accepts Aetna Insurance" and getting only those searches that use that exact phrase, or something very close to it.

The broader your search, the wider your marketing message will reach, but the less targeted it will be. Test the various match types to keep whittling your list down to find the most viable keywords that will give you the best results for your ad budget.

Searching for New Keywords

To search for ad groups and keywords from scratch, click on the tab 'Search for New Keyword and Ad Group Ideas' within the Keyword Planner dashboard.

Keyword Planner
Plan your next search campaign

What would you like to do?

    ▸ **Search for new keyword and ad group ideas**

Here you are encouraged to tell Google a little bit about your products and services.

▾ **Search for new keyword and ad group ideas**

Enter one or more of the following:

Your product or service

For example, flowers or used cars

Your landing page

www.example.com/page

Your product category

Enter or select a product category

Start with a phrase that not only describes your practice, but that also separates you from all the other professionals of your kind optimizing for similar keywords. Remember to use geographic modifiers, such as, "Austin Cosmetic Dentistry" or "General Dentistry in Beverly Hills".

Next, enter the URL of your practice's website and a category that is relevant to your practice. As with most Google products of this type, the moment you start typing your category, Google will try to predict what you are trying to say. Choose your categories based on the suggestions you are given, as those are usually the most searched for within the Adwords system.

At the bottom of this initial form, you will notice a spot to indicate a number of filters you might like to use to narrow your keyword research down even further. You can select the country, language and network to search for, as well as enter negative keywords so as not to waste your time.

Use the filters as you see fit, such as only searching keywords that enjoy more than 100 searches per month or only those keywords that offer at least 1000 impressions for the advertisers who are optimizing for them. You can include words, exclude words and basically customize your search however you prefer.

When you are satisfied with your criteria, hit the button Get Ideas and you will be taken to the Keyword Results page.

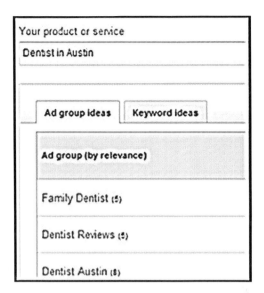

At the top of the Keyword Results page is a tab where you can select Ad Group ideas and Keyword ideas.

Ad group ideas will provide you with the most popular ad groups in your category, a list of the most popular keywords within those ad groups, as well as other vital information.

Average Monthly Searches: This number lets you know just how popular that ad group or keyword happens to be. The higher the number, the more popular the term tends to be, and the more competition it is likely to have.

Competition: This represents the level of competition the ad group or keyword enjoys in three increments: Low, Medium and High. The lower the competition level, the easier it will be for your practice to rank for the ad groups and keywords you plan to optimize for.

Suggested Bid: No more guessing how much to bid and hoping that your ads show up for relevant searches. This number takes into account all the other advertisers bidding for that keyword, and yields a monthly total that will give you a leg up in the keyword bidding war; particularly if your competitors fail to use the Keyword Planner tool.

Ad Impression Share: This number takes into account your location and chosen ad network and yields the likelihood of that keyword receiving impressions and clicks. When you see a high percentage, click on the Add to Plan button to put that ad group or keyword into a separate planning compartment, similar to an ecommerce shopping cart.

Monthly Searches: If you look closely, there is an icon that looks like a tiny graph directly in front of the search number. Hover over it and you will be able to view the average search volume for that ad group or keyword over the past few months. This is perfect for identifying trends that may be experiencing an uphill swing that you can then take advantage of.

Add to Plan: Here you can implement new ad group ideas, remove them and edit them before you incorporate them into a campaign that will soon be or that is currently running.

When you have successfully put together a plan that you are sure will give your dental Internet marketing campaign a boost, click on the button Review Estimates.

Keyword Planner Estimates and Review Plan

New Ad Groups and Keywords

This section allows you to see the clicks, cost and impressions per day that the ad group or keyword experiences, as well as other details like the average position on the search results page and the overall cost to your Adwords budget.

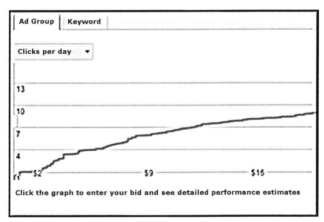

You can search, test and upload as an Excel or CSV file any ad groups or keywords that you wish to examine.

Existing Keyword Lists

Earlier you brainstormed and compiled a list of dental keywords and you have been using those terms throughout your basic and advanced Internet marketing campaigns. This is the section of the Keyword Planner where you can copy and paste your list or upload it as a CSV file to check its viability.

> ▸ Get search volume for a list of keywords or group them into ad groups

Don't forget to list your keywords naked (Broad search), with quotes (Phrase search) or with brackets (Exact search) so that you get the most accurate results for your needs.

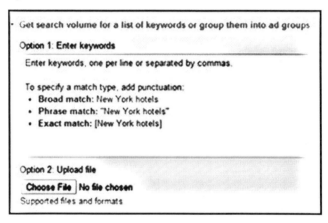

When you are finished, click Get Volume to proceed to the results page.

To estimate the amounts of traffic that you are likely to experience with your existing list of keywords, click on the link 'Get traffic estimates for a list of keywords'.

> ▸ **Get traffic estimates for a list of keywords**

Again, enter your keywords naked, in brackets or quotes, or upload them as a CSV file and then hit Get Estimates to continue.

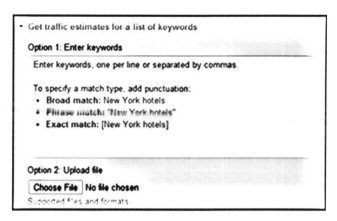

Mixing and Matching for New Ideas

To combine and multiply your keywords, click on the menu item 'Multiply keyword lists to get new keyword ideas'. This allows you to combine your current keywords together.

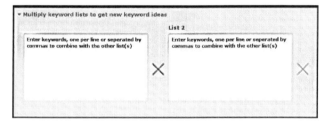

Simply enter the first keyword you want combined, such as Dentistry in Austin, with a secondary keyword that you want that keyword combined with, such as Cosmetic Dentistry in Texas.

When you are finished, click on Click on Get Estimates or Get Search Volume to see the respective results.

You are encouraged to use the Keyword Planner to get new keyword ideas and to narrow down your existing lists until you find those highly-sought after keyword terms that no one or that only a few other professionals of your ilk are pursuing.

Once you have a list of keywords that you know are well-performing, or that you are sure to get conversions out of, go back and start plugging those keywords into your on and off-site SEO campaigns, use them on your social media profiles and in your email marketing campaigns.

Then keep the keyword research ongoing so that you can keep up with trends, buyer preferences and current Adwords data.

Advanced PPC Marketing – The Possibilities

With your first Adwords campaign running, you should start receiving clicks to your website, blog and social media accounts or anywhere else you have provided links to. Over time, and after enough data has flowed in, you will be able to identify certain advertising trends. Like we mentioned before, you might begin to notice that most of your ad traffic is coming from tablet computers. Likewise, you may notice that most of your traffic happens between nine in the morning until twelve in the afternoon and only on weekdays.

As an Adwords advertiser, you have many variables at your disposal that you can use to further hone your advertising skills and more massively stretch your advertising budget. You can set your ads to run at certain times of the day, in certain areas, you can rotate ads and test them. You can run reports, set data filters and tweak your ads until they are bringing in the traffic and leads that you expect.

And remember, there are also display ads, different Google networks and other variables that we haven't even begun to explore. For now, we have provided you with the basics of setting up your first campaign and now your Internet marketing net is almost complete.

You have a website, a blog, a social media presence, an email marketing campaign and now a paid Internet marketing campaign. With your net established, you should be trapping leads left and right, enticing them to call, email and visit; and at the same time, you should be capturing those leads' information and converting them using the staff training lessons we discussed in the very beginning.

The only thing left to do now is test and tweak your approach to deliver even more results. If the phone is ringing and the lobby is filling up, prepare to expand your practice even more. You might even need a bigger building, and growing your practice to earn $5 million per year is just the way to get it.

Chapter 12: Tracking Your Efforts, Analytics, Acquisition Cost Analysis and ROI

This is the section of the book where we determine how well all the various parts of your Internet marketing campaign are performing. You will find out which of your web pages are getting the most attention and why, how much you are spending to acquire each new patient and where your Internet marketing budget is most paying off.

The first thing we do when you want to measure the performance of a particular campaign is identify one or more KPIs or Key Performance Indicators.

Step 1: Establish Key Performance Indicators

In marketing – both online and offline – a KPI is any measurable element that determines the effectiveness of any aspect of a particular campaign. Consider the following examples, which you may set as KPIs for your own practice.

- The amount of traffic that lands on your individual practice web pages.
- The amount of people that land on various pages after finding your site link on social media.
- The number of leads that call after finding a phone number on your website.
- The website forms that people use to send communications to your office.

Think of your KPIs as your marketing results from click to call, though we are also interested in those patients that email or that visit in the flesh-and-blood. For KPIs to have any significance, you first need to be able to track your results.

have seen a tiny bit of this tracking in your Adwords dashboard. Google kes it easy to determine which ads are performing by providing you with alytics data the moment you log in.

You are going to now further track your results by using another free tool – Google Analytics – as well as some other tactics that will help you set and measure the KPIs you wish to track.

In the beginning you are going to have all this data coming in, which will seem like nothing more than numbers and figures at first. Soon, however, you will begin to notice trends and patterns and you will then be able to use those patterns to hone your marketing messages and improve your overall results.

***

Step 2: Track All Phone Calls

Before we even began discussing dental Internet marketing, we prepared your practice for receiving phone calls from interested prospects, current patients and former patients alike. The reasoning that we gave you at the time was that, with all of these Internet marketing steps, the phone would soon begin ringing off the hook. Well, if you have followed along up to this point, the phone should be ringing. Now it is time to discover just where your results paid off enough to cause interested parties to pick up the phone and give your practice a ring.

Why We Advise Against Call Tracking Phone Numbers

Phone call trackers are automated programs that allow you to detect who is calling, what time they called and exactly what was said. In some cases, you can have the conversation printed out into an easy-to-analyze text document.

Google Voice is a good example of a call tracker. You can use your own phone number or you can get a Google Voice phone number that you get to choose (as long as the number is available). You can opt to receive a Google Voice number that includes your local area code, for example.

Call trackers like these are great and they offer tons of data that can be analyzed to further improve your marketing efforts, but they can also hurt your local search rankings.

Earlier we mentioned that local SERPs were largely supplied from the big three data aggregators, yellow page sites and other directories; and you spent a lot of time ensuring that the information on those platforms was accurate and consistent.

Many of those platforms look to determine if the phone number you use is consistent with the address you list as your practice location. If the phone number and address don't jive, the platforms – and particularly Google – will think that you are trying to game the system. This could drop you down a few notches in the local SERPs or it could take you off the first page altogether. Just a word of warning.

Instead of using call trackers, we recommend that you train your staff to ask every caller how they heard of the practice and where they received the phone number. We also recommended recording phone calls to ensure that the proper phone policies are being followed.

You might leave a prospect form by each phone with a special place for staff to enter where the prospect found the office phone number. You will then be able to determine where to put most of your Internet marketing efforts, such as if most of your prospects are calling from the website, and where to improve your efforts, such as if little to no calls are originating from social media.

Don't just train staff to ask for the location; instruct them to data mine however possible. For instance, if a caller says that they found the phone number on your website, ask how they found the website. If the caller found the site through Google, ask him/her what keyword terms were used to conduct the search.

You may also ask callers to identify how they found the practice on the outgoing answering message and you might leave instructions with the answering service to data mine this information, if the practice uses one.

Only by tracking phone calls can you accurately set and assess your KPIs as they relate to all telephone calls coming into your practice from your Internet marketing efforts.

***

Step 3: Set Up Google Analytics

This is Google's platform that we mentioned that will allow you to track nearly every KPI that you establish and wish to track. You can track your website traffic, social media accounts, email marketing campaigns and Adwords PPC campaigns all from a single dashboard.

First you need to tell Analytics about your website so that it can start recording your site's traffic and conversions. There are two ways to access Analytics. You can visit the Google Analytics sign in page by visiting www.Google.com/analytics and clicking on Access Analytics; or you can go to your Adwords account, then select Tools and Analytics from the drop down menu.

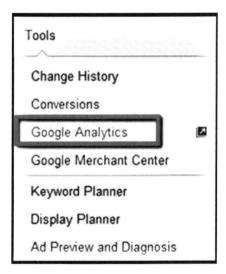

Both methods will allow you to sign up and start using the web data tracking platform right away.

How to Install Analytics on your WordPress Website

After you have signed into Analytics, you will be asked to select a few preferences. When you are asked about the type of account that you would like to track, select Website. Google Analytics will also allow you to track the web data for mobile apps, but for right now you are only interested in tracking the web data that is associated with your practice's website.

For the tracking method, we suggest Universal Analytics, which offers the broadest range of options. You will also have access to future Analytics updates and features.

Now you are ready to set up your account. Choose your Account Name, which is a title of your choosing, the name of your practice's website, the

URL of your website, your business category – we suggest Healthcare – and your reporting time zone.

The data sharing settings are up to you. The more check boxes you select, the more data Google will glean over time and the better Analytics should become. When you have made your selections, check Get Tracking ID and move on to the next step.

Installing Your Tracking Code

The snippet of code that you are provided with in the next section is designed to be placed into the internal workings of your website. Since you are using WordPress, placing your Analytics code into your website is as easy as finding the place and copying and pasting it in.

First, visit your WordPress website's dashboard, select Appearance on the left hand pane and then find the Editor button.

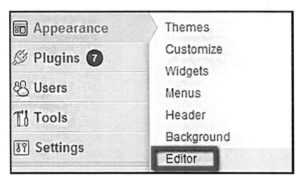

Inside the Editor, find the Header link on the right hand side of your screen and click on it to expand it. This will show you and allow you to edit the code that is included in the Header section of your WordPress website.

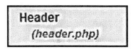

Find the </body> tag and copy and paste your snippet of code directly above that tag. Be sure to leave a space between the tag and the snippet of code for easy finding and editing later.

An even easier method is to go to Plugins, then Add New to search for the WordPress Analytics plugin. You will only need to insert your Analytics ID number, which is provided on the same page as the snippet of code and starts with UA followed by a series of numbers.

When you are finished with either step, refresh the Tracking Code page and you should see a message that reads, "Tracking Installed". That is when you know that Google Analytics is tracking and reporting successfully.

Important KPIs to Track with Analytics

Your Analytics dashboard may seem a bit bare at first, but you will be provided with all sorts of data once your individual Internet marketing campaigns have received consistent attention. You can customize your dashboard any way you would like so that it displays any data you prefer, but the default data will work perfectly for now. In one glance, you should be able to determine some or all of the following.

Search Times: Analytics allows you to view the traffic you are receiving to your website by the month, week, day or hour. By determining when most of your traffic seems to flow, you can concentrate your marketing efforts to coincide with those very times. For example, you may find that Saturdays and Sundays – which typically enjoy the most click-through-rates – are really hot for social media referrals; so you may choose to keep a staff member on-hand and social-media-active during those times.

Site/Page Visits: Most marketers are immediately interested in the overall amount of visitors that land on their site, but dig a bit deeper and see which of your individual pages are landed on the most. If you notice that one or more of your pages are receiving more page visits than others, find out what those pages have that the others lack and alter your approach accordingly.

External Referral Sources: This metric determines how well you happen to be doing in your off-site SEO efforts. By determining where most of your traffic originates from – other websites, social media profiles, directories, blog posts or plain old Google SERPs – you can then focus your future off-site SEO efforts on those platforms; since you now know how hot they are for lead generation.

Time on Site/Page: In a perfect world, everyone who landed on our site would stay a while, browse around, watch your videos, write down your phone number and use your contact form; resulting in an average stay of at least five minutes. The reality is that most visitors will remain on your site for about a minute, some more, some less. Take a look at those pages that seem to keep visitors around and attempt to replicate those elements for the pages that don't enjoy such a high retention rate. You may have to make your site colors easier to view, your content easier to read or your contact forms easier to submit. The longer you can manage to keep visitors on your site, the more likely they are to become interested and convert.

Bounce Rate: As the term suggests, this is the amount of people who land on your site and then immediately click away. They may click back to the search results or they may click another link, but the general message is the same: Your site simply did not have what the visitor was looking for. By studying the bounce rate of your individual pages, you can determine what would make someone want to leave.

Some searchers may have entered wrong terms, which is why negative keywords are recommended for your PPC account. For example, a searcher looking for Dental Implants Manufacturers may click on your Dental Implants services page by mistake. Your job is to make sure that your ads don't show up for Implants manufacturers.

You may find that your site looks too cheap or that your web copy contains errors and misspellings or that your photos are blurry or that your videos simply will not play. All of these issues can be fixed and your site's bounce rate will help to draw your attention to them.

Keywords & Phrases: For those prospects and patients who did happen find your site via the search engines, Analytics will tell you exactly which keywords were used most often to find your individual pages. This can help you determine new viable keywords - and negative keywords - to improve all of your Internet marketing campaigns.

External Analytics Platforms

Google analytics is useful for tracking an immense amount of data from your website, but there are other analytics platforms that we want to draw your attention to right now. By gleaning and analyzing all the data you can get your hands on, you can obtain a more accurate snapshot of how well your campaigns are performing.

Email Tracking: Your Mail Chimp email marketing platform comes with a built-in analytics mechanism that will allow you track data related to your subscriber audience and the level of engagement that you experience with that audience. You can see, in real-time, how many people have opened your emails, who has clicked links within the emails and which subscribers are completely non-responsive.

As luck or innovation would have it, Mail Chimp now allows you to merge your Mail Chimp account with your Google Analytics account. Simply find the button to connect the two in your Mail Chimp settings and you will begin to receive email marketing data immediately. This information can then be seamlessly merged with your other analytics data to determine how your multiple campaigns are performing with a single glance of your Google Analytics dashboard.

Social Media Tracking: Many social media platforms also offer analytics capabilities to their users. Facebook Insights, Twitter Analytics and YouTube Analytics are a few examples. This data allows you to determine which of your posts are receiving the most attention, which are shared with other network users and which media elements are being passed around the most.

***

Step 4: Run Regular Analytics Reports

We recommend that you run, retain and study regular reports - weekly, monthly or every three months – to accurately assess where your Internet marketing results are most paying off. This will require the help of your staff members to gauge phone calls, emails and visitors that walk-in through the door. Track everything, online and off, to determine what works and what doesn't. Then improve on what is working to bring even more well-paying patients into your office.

***

Step 5: Track Patient Online Behavior

When the phone does ring, it is your hope that any staff member who answers the phone will be able to close the caller right away, as in make the person a brand new patient. Whether the sale is closed or not, the results of the call or other interaction should always be recorded and analyzed so that the life of the patient can be tracked from the point of initial interest all the way to the act of paying for the first of many dental appointments.

In the act of doing so, you may detect patterns forming. For instance, you may find that most of your patients are locating your website through Facebook and then calling your practice from your website. By understanding these associations, you can focus your energy and efforts to improve the amounts of leads that are received and closed.

***

Step 6: Calculate Your Patient Lifetime Value

We are a fan of tracking everything you can get your hands on; and understanding the lifetime value (LTV) of each of your patients is, in our opinion, the best way to track your overall return on investment (ROI). Not only that, but your LTV will also help you set the most advantageous marketing budget when it comes to Adwords or other paid Internet marketing platforms.

To calculate the total lifetime value of your patients, identify the following values.

Average Treatment Value (ATV): Take the total amount your practice earns and divide that number by the amount of treatments your practice performs each year.

Average Treatments Per Patient Per Year (ATP): Take the total number of treatments that your practice performs each year and divide that number by the amount of patients your practice serves to calculate the ATP.

Patient Duration: This is the amount of time, in years, that the average patient remains active in your database.

Average Number of Referrals Per Year: This number is calculated a bit differently.

No referrals is characterized by the single digit 1.

2 referrals in 20 patients or 1 in 5 (20%) is calculated as 1.2.

5 referrals in 10 patients or 1 in 2 (50%) is calculated as 1.5, and so on.

Now multiply those variables together. For instance, your ATV may be $100, your ATP might be 2, your patient duration may be 5 years and your average referral rate may be 1.4. Calculating that amount, you will find a patient lifetime value of $1,400.

This information becomes useful when you have a specific goal in mind, say like becoming a $5 million practice like Mint Dental has done. This figure also helps you determine how well your Internet marketing campaigns may be performing.

If you didn't know this figure and you earned 3 new patients through Internet marketing, you might assume that three patients times $100 for the

181

average treatment value only contributes $300 to the practice overall. A low figure like that can contribute to feeling discouraged if your goal is a lofty $5 million or more.

On the other hand, when you know that each patient contributes $1,400 to your practice, three new patients will yield $4, 200, If you can manage to analyze your data and tweak your campaigns accordingly to double or even quadruple your lead gains, three new patients could end up contributing $25,200, $50,400 and so on.

When you look at the situation like that, setting a goal of earning $5 million per year doesn't seem that far away at all.

***

Step 7: Calculate Your Return on Investment (ROI)

Once you know the lifetime value of each patient you earn, you are now in a better position to calculate the amount of return your practice earns on your marketing investment. Let's assume that you spend $5,000 total on a domain name, hosting, advanced Mail Chimp functionality and an Adwords account with dozens of ads running in constant rotation.

To calculate your rate of return, you will take the amount of new patients that you have earned from your campaign and multiply that number by the LTV that you calculated above. Subtract that number from your Internet marketing investment and divide that number by your Internet marketing investment.

So your formula may look like this:

((New Patients * LTV) – Investment)
Investment

For example, if you earn 12 new patients through your Internet marketing efforts and you earn an LTV of $1,400 per year per patient, and you spend $5,000 on your Internet marketing efforts, your rate of return would be 2.36%.

We recommend that you set up another tab in your Internet marketing spreadsheet to track your patient acquisition costs and rate of return, along with all of your other report data.

***

Step 8: Set Marketing Goals

We discussed setting marketing goals in the section where you created your Internet marketing plan. We ask that you return to that section now and use the information you have learned in the meantime to fortify and further expand your overall marketing campaign. This includes both your basic and advanced Internet marketing efforts.

Based on your market, keyword and competitor research, start to formulate steps that you would need to take to reach your goal of earning $5 million per year.

A typical campaign may look like this.

GenericDental bills on average $3,000,000 per year to its patients, has 1200 patients, an average treatment rate of 6, an average patient duration of 4 years and a referral rate of 1.2. Thus the practice earns about $12,000 per new patient.

If GenericDental wants to earn $5 million per year, the practice will need to earn 167 new patients in a single year. This may seem like a lofty number, but it's not once you realize that it's only 14 new patients per month or 3.5 new patients per week.

Since GenericDental is located in a large metropolitan area, this goal doesn't seem impossible at all. To recruit those 3.5 new patients, GenericDental puts the following action plan into effect:

- 3 new blog posts published every week
- 10 Facebook, Twitter and Google+ posts per week
- 1 new video posted on YouTube per month
- 1 email newsletter sent per month
- 12 PPC ad groups running in rotation that coincide with the practice's services with 5 ads running in each group.

Having a set patient goal in mind will help you establish a series of dental Internet marketing goals that will help you meet your primary recruitment goal.

For right now, until data starts rolling in, set up your website and start publishing a few blogs per month. Don't forget to watch out for and respond to comments when they come in. Then start posting to social media and send out your first of many email marketing messages. Establish a PPC account and keep an eye on your analytics figures.

Then tell your staff about your recruitment goals so that everyone is on the same page. Make a contest out of it and ensure that your staff members have fun while they do their best to help you build your practice from the ground up. As the phone rings, as emails come in and as the door chimes go off with each new person that strolls into your lobby, your practice should begin to operating like a well-oiled machine.

***

Step 9: Test & Tweak to Improve Conversions

Rarely do Internet marketers get everything perfect right out of the gate, despite how much research they may have been conducted beforehand. This is why studying your analytics figures is so vital to your overall marketing success. Your figures will tell you what is working, what is not so effective and you can respond in kind to make your campaigns even better.

A/B Testing

This is a technique used by Internet marketers to improve campaigns that involves two similar elements that are tweaked slightly in the hopes of delivering measurable results. For example, imagine that you have an Adwords ad that is performing slightly well, but you are not seeing quite as much traffic as you would like.

To test the ad, you will comprise a duplicate ad that will run at the same time of day to the exact same audience, but possibly on alternating days. The difference is that the second ad will have a slightly different headline. By testing the two headlines with the same audience, you can determine which one is more effective at enticing prospects to click. You can then keep that headline and test the body of the ad, for example, then the landing page that you send your click-throughs to, and so on.

Testing is time consuming, particularly when you take into account the fact that you must let your test subjects sit in order to collect data. Whatever you do, don't become impatient and stop your testing early to tweak another aspect of your ad, blog or other element. You must handle your testing like a scientist. Change one variable, keep everything else consistent, tabulate the results and then start again until every element has been analyzed – and optimized.

After enough time has passed and enough testing has been conducted, you will find those elements that your audience truly responds to, and your results will speak for themselves.

Improving Conversions

After a while you will be obsessed with converting your prospects and patients at every turn; when they call the practice, come in to check out the office, send an online form, click on an ad, read one of your blog posts or watch a video on one of your webpages.

With enough attention, research and after getting to know your audience, the elements you need to change and the avenues you need to pursue will become clear as day.

But what if things don't quite work as you expect? When you need a little help with your campaigns, it is important to have an Internet marketing troubleshooting guide; which we have provided for you in the very next section.

Chapter 13: Troubleshooting Your Internet Marketing Campaigns

If your campaigns seem to be floundering, if web traffic isn't quite coming your way or if your visitors seem to bounce more often than not, it is important to keep the following troubleshooting cheat sheet close by. Here are the three most common symptoms for why your Internet marketing campaigns aren't performing and how to fix them to keep the conversions coming.

Symptom #1: Help, my website is fine but my traffic levels are really low.

Possible Fixes:

1. Search for your keywords in Google to determine where your site is ranking in the search results. Click on the other sites that are outranking you to determine what elements you can emulate to boost your rankings.
2. Ensure that you are targeting long-tail keywords and phrases along with geographic location modifiers, particularly in your website title tags, headlines and sub-headlines.
3. Use a responsive design or a dedicated mobile site so that mobile device users get the web experience they are intended to receive.
4. Run a Yext and/or Whitespark report to determine if your citations listed across the web are accurate and consistent.
5. Publish a new blog post at least once per week to keep your content fresh.
6. Run a PPC campaign that focuses on your local market.
7. Check that all of the links that point to your site are working properly and that they contain hypertext (the words that make up the link) that is relevant to the page visitors will be landing on. For

example, a link that reads Dental Implants should only point to a page that discusses dental implants.

***

Symptom #2: My traffic levels are fine, but I'm not getting as many calls, emails or office visits as I expected.

Possible Fixes:

1. Check the call-to-actions that are listed on your website and individual pages. Determine if they could be stronger or more targeted to the actions you are expecting visitors to take.

2. Fill out one of your own contact forms to see if you receive any errors and to ensure that all of your messages are getting through.

3. Click on every one of your website pages to ensure that they are working. While you are at it, check all links pointing to your site as well as internal links to ensure that they are whole, complete and leading visitors to the intended landing pages.

4. WordPress sites are intended to show up perfectly for pretty much all web browsers. The actual theme you choose may be a different story. Check your site in Chrome, Firefox and Internet Explorer to determine if all of your visitors are receiving the intended experience.

5. Check your content to ensure that it is targeted and of the highest-quality. Make sure all of your visitors are able to find exactly what they are searching for when clicking on your site and individual pages.

6. Run analytics reports to see which of your pages, blogs, ads and other marketing messages are converting and where you can possibly improve things.

7. You may try placing a section on your website that reads 'Why Choose Us?' along with several bullet points that describe your practice's primary benefits. In our experience, this can really help with website conversions.

8. Place your practice specials and discounts right on your home page and above the fold so that visitors don't have to search to find it.

9. Ensure that you have trust logos right on your home page. These don't have to be above the fold, but they should be present if you hope to gain extra credibility.

10. All in all, ensure that your visitors have an easy and stress-free user experience. You may even get a few opinions from trusted patients to determine possible fixes that could help your conversions improve.

***

Symptom #3: Emails are coming in and the phone is ringing, but those prospects aren't turning into actual appointments.

1. Ensure that the staff is properly trained and that all staff members who answer the phones are following the agreed-upon phone protocol.
2. Record your office phone calls and listen for anything that may be hindering the conversion process.
3. Train staff members to check and respond to practice emails regularly and to always use calls-to-action that cause prospects to call, submit or visit.
4. Follow a lead nurturing schedule that has your staff members calling leads on a regular basis. If you need extra incentive to do so, consider the studies that show that nurtured leads make 47% larger purchases than non-nurtured leads. In dental circles, that means more premium treatments that further expand your bottom line.

Chapter 14: The Future of Your Practice Is Now In Your Hands

Congratulations for getting through this crash course in dental Internet marketing! If you were reading with the intentions of going back through to put this advice into action, you now have a much better understanding of how dental professionals get found on the web.

If you have been working this entire time to put your Internet marketing plan into action, not only do you have a better understanding of search engine optimization and most things digital, but you may also be experiencing actual results.

If you have been following and working along, you now have a website that is optimized for local search results using well-researched keywords, metadata, useful content and strong calls-to-action.

You have an active blog that provides even more fresh content to your hungry audience.

You have active social media accounts where you take part in conversations, help out when necessary and further spread your content to all four corners of the Internet.

You have an email marketing campaign that regularly ships out useful advice in concise messages that also include strong calls-to-action.

You have a PPC marketing campaign that is well-tested and regularly monitored in order to improve conversions.

And all the while you are running regular analytics reports and constantly tweaking your campaigns from site to ad in order to maximize the amounts of clicks, calls, emails and visits your practice experiences on a daily basis.

If you have done all of those things up to this point, you deserve a big pat on the back. You are well on your way to owning and operating a $5 million practice. There are two ways that we recommend proceeding from here.

Option A

We advise you to take what you have learned in this book and apply the steps bit-by-bit and piece-by-piece, doing most of the work yourself while delegating what you can to your staff.

Option B

You can take what you have learned in this book to approach an organization comprised of professionals who can handle all of the heavy Internet marketing lifting for you.

Here is why we recommend the latter option for your dental practice.

Your practice is far too busy to introduce a series of extra steps like social media posting, email marketing, blog writing, responding to comments and ad creation thrown into the mix. This will become especially true when your Internet marketing efforts start coming to fruition.

A successful practice requires the full focus of everyone involved – dentists, technicians, front desk staff, office managers and everyone else who may be involved in your day-to-days. That is why we recommend the services of a professional Internet marketing company that can deliver the skills, training and resources your practice needs to be successful online, while keeping you aware of your progress every step of the way.

That is what worked for Mint Dental and all the other dental offices we have helped through the years, and we recommend the same course of action for you. If you want to reach your goal of earning $5 million each and every year, you now have the know-how and steps; you just have to act. Whether you do it on your own or with a group by your side, your dental office will flourish. Here is to your success. We wish you all that you desire and more.

About the Authors

Adam Zilko and Jacob Puhl are friends, ambitious business leaders and co-owners of Firegang Digital Marketing. Since the two first met Jake and Adam have strived to remain at the forefront of the Internet marketing industry.

Despite the fact that Jake runs his office in Cincinnati, Ohio and Adam does the same in Anchorage, Alaska, the two have combined their efforts to form and grow one of the most competitive digital marketing organizations of our day.

The two can usually be found studying some aspect of the industry, networking with others in exciting new fields and assisting dental professionals with their ever-growing desire to dominate their local online marketplaces.

The two regularly perform at public speaking engagements, are keen on traveling and meeting with top dignitaries in their field and their primary interest is in helping all dental professionals reach their practice goals.

About Firegang Digital Marketing

Firegang has existed in one form or another since the early 2000's. A digital marketing company with offices in Cincinnati, Ohio; Anchorage, Alaska; and Spokane, Washington, the company provides small to medium sized businesses with the edge they need to get ahead online.

From web design to content creation to paid online advertising campaigns to regular reports to showcase all results, Firegang provides personalized service that is tailored specifically for the company in question; and the results speak for themselves.

The company began by helping SMBs in all industries, but for the last few years, and after a string of successful campaigns for dental professionals all across the US, Firegang has been focused on learning the intricacies of Dental Internet Marketing.

The company regularly publishes Digital Dental Magazine, an online resource for dentists, dental staff, marketers and consultants; which provides tips, tricks and inside secrets to getting dental practices found online.

To learn more about Firegang, to send a message to the authors or to receive a free analysis and quote on any future or existing Internet marketing campaigns, email Admin@Firegang.com.

Made in the USA
Lexington, KY
16 June 2014